THE NURSE AND HER **PROBLEM**
PATIENTS

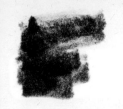

THE NURSE AND HER
PROBLEM
PATIENTS

by GERTRUD BERTRAND UJHELY, R.N., M.A.
*Assistant Professor of Nursing, Rutgers, the State University of
New Jersey*

SPRINGER Publishing Company, Inc., New York

First printing, May 1963
Second printing, September 1965
Third printing, April 1967

Library of Congress Catalog Card Number: 63-11842

Printed in U.S.A.

TO MY
FATHER AND MOTHER
IN GRATITUDE

PREFACE

Some readers may wonder why there should be a book on the nurse and her problem patients: "Does not the author know that there are no problem patients but only problem nurses?" I think we cannot be so categorical as that. Any nurse, and her supervisor, will recognize that the conscientious nurse practitioner, whose duties are constant and continuous, will at times focus on the "problem" most obvious and urgent to her—the patient who "interferes with her work." And these, of course, become the problem patients. The hard-pressed, overworked nurse—and every nurse is that, some days or everyday—needs, and should expect, help with her problem patients, help that may enable her in time to evaluate her own part in these difficulties and that may contribute to modifying her own outlook and behavior accordingly. This book has been written with the intention of offering such help.

Some readers may ask, why another book on nurse-patient relationships. I believe that most of the books already in print, though well worth reading, do not present the problems in the way that most nurse practitioners perceive them. Instead, the books proceed in a fashion imposed by one or another theoretical framework. I believe, further, that unless the nurse is helped to coordinate the theoretical material with the problems she perceives, she may not be able to make full use of even the best text on interpersonal relations.

The theory presented and developed comes from many sources. Some of it is derived from what I have absorbed in my four years' association with Hildegard E. Peplau, R.N., Ed.D., and her students, at Rutgers University. Some is based on my training in the profession, my reading, and the teach-ings of my psychotherapists. I have attempted to acknowledge sources wherever pertinent, but much of what I have learned has become so much a part of me that it is difficult to trace it back to the various original sources.

This book focuses on the nurse and her difficulties with patients. Since it is not an exhaustive treatise but an expression of my own thinking, it will supplement pre-service or in-service teaching rather than replace it. The book gives answers, but it also raises questions, some of which the reader will be able to answer herself, in time.

The nurse and her problem patients is written primarily for the practitioner in nursing and the nursing student who take care of adult patients in the general hospital. Implications can be drawn for the nursing of patients in clinical specialties such as obstetrics, pediatrics, psychiatry, public health, or the care of patients with long-term diseases.

Since the book deals with problem situations, it pays little attention to the nurse for whom such situations are not problems. I do not mean to imply that all nurses have problems with all or any of the situations outlined here. Since there are more female than male nurses, I have used the feminine pronoun in the book when referring to nurses.

New York,   GERTRUD B. UJHELY
January 1963

ACKNOWLEDGMENTS

I would like to make acknowledgment to various friends and colleagues, for although this subject has been in my mind for many years, it would not have reached bookform without the help and encouragement of others. My father's casual remark that he saw no reason why I could not write a book, reminded me of Dr. Emma Spaney's earlier and more specific suggestion. Miss Dorothy W. Smith, R.N., Ed.D., encouraged me to enlarge upon the ideas presented when I was a consultant for a chapter on interpersonal relationships in her textbook *Care of the Adult Patient,* written jointly with Miss Claudia D. Gips, R.N., Ed.D.

Miss Peplau, of Rutgers, repeatedly urged me to put my thoughts in writing and helped me to organize the preliminary outline of the book. Miss Phyllis Hurteau, R.N., B.S., and Miss Elsa Poslusny, R.N., M.A., gave many hours of their time in listening to entire chapters. They made valuable suggestions concerning content and source materials, and offered persistent encouragement especially at times when the going was difficult.

Miss Joyce Crane, R.N., M.S., Miss Anne C. David, M.A., M.S.W., Miss M. Lucille Murphy, R.N., M.A., Miss Ann Nunnencamp, Mrs. Nancy Sarsfield, R.N., M.A., Mrs. Esther Schattman, M.A., Miss Smith, Miss Joan Walsh, R.N., M.Ed., and Miss Leona Weiner, R.N., M.A., have each read or listened to selected chapters and have been generous with their advice when questioned about factual material.

Miss Gips read various drafts of the manuscript critically for its effect on readers and made many invaluable suggestions concerning organization, clarity, tone of content, and choice of examples.

Miss Frances Purdy, R.N., M.Litt., offered to open her clinical facilities to me in the event that I needed validation from her staff. Dean Frances Reiter, R.N., M.A., of the Graduate School,

New York Medical College, made it possible for me to consult with members of the clinical staff regarding certain areas. Miss Mary Hussey, R.N., M.A., contributed some clinical data.

The graduate nurses who participated in the workshops on problem patients and the undergraduate students of the College of Nursing at Rutgers not only furnished me with many insights concerning the relationship between nurses and their problem patients but also repeatedly expressed their need for a discussion of this subject in written form.

Miss Pat Pollak, A.B., was generous in offering to type several chapters of the book.

Finally, I would like to thank my friends who did not withdraw their interest in spite of my lack of time for socializing in the past year.

I wish to stress, in conclusion, that, although I gratefully acknowledge the help I received in making this book a reality, the responsibility for its contents rests entirely and exclusively with me.   **G. B. U.**

CONTENTS

PART III:
Some Solutions to Having Problem Patients

INTRODUCTION

Problem patients are familiar to nurses, despite the fact that most nurses and their supervisors have probably tried to persuade themselves that there are no such people. It's not the patient who is the problem—it's the nurse; just as there are no problem children, merely problem parents. However, this generality is too simple, and of no particular use. It is helpful to recognize that many a parent has found some solution for his own problems after he has become aware of his children's problems, and when he has sought help for them. Similarly, the nurse practitioner sees first the problem patients, and then realizes that it is primarily her job, not the patient's, to cope with, and understand, the difficulty.

In the meantime the patients who hold up the flow of work by obstructing it with their demands, complaints, or lack of cooperation will continue to arouse the anger of the nurse. Other patients who because of their age, cultural background, or the nature of their illness do not respond sufficiently to the nurse's ministrations may continue to arouse emotions in her which can range from hopelessness to guilt to helpless rage. All or any one of these emotions also make it more difficult for the nurse to do her work adequately. It is understandable that, in order to free herself emotionally for her work, the nurse will go on labeling the patient with adjectives that put the blame on him.

The categories of problem patients discussed in this book were selected because, it became apparent to me, there are certain recurrent problem situations between nurses and patients. These I have noted in my personal experiences as staff nurse in general hospitals, from questionnaires answered

1

by hundreds of nursing students and graduate practitioners, from seminars with students and workshops with graduates, from the data of two studies ((1, 2),* and from the literature (3,4,5). Interestingly enough, patients who required complicated procedures in their nursing care were not labeled as "difficult" or "problem" patients in any of the returned questionnaires or in any of the discussion groups. I have selected the most commonly occurring problem situations: those that most frequently turn up in answered questionnaires, in nurses' reports at the change of shifts, and those for which students and graduate nurses most frequently ask for help in seminars and workshops.

The book is divided into three parts. It begins with a discussion of why nurses may be having problem patients in the first place. Then it deals with the problems and explores some specific reasons for their existence and some possibilities for their solution. The last part is a discussion of some of the general issues raised in the first part, with suggested ways of solving them.

Suggested Reading

Some texts on interpersonal relations for nurses or useful to them:

Talking With Patients, by Brian Bird (Lippincott, 1955) .

Personal, Impersonal, and Interpersonal Relations, by Genevieve Burton (Springer, 1958).

The Dynamic Nurse-Patient Relationship, by Ida Jean Orlando (Putnam, 1961).

Interpersonal Relations in Nursing, by Hildegard E. Peplau (Putnam, 1952). This is not written in easy language, but it is worth a try.

---

* See Notes at the end of the book for all sources referred to by number, as above.

PART I

WHY DOES THE NURSE HAVE PROBLEM PATIENTS?

Chapter 1
The Nurse May Have Unrealistic Expectations of Herself

Before getting into a discussion of the kinds of patients whom nurses consider to be "problem" patients, it may be worthwhile to consider some of the reasons why, at least in my opinion, nurses have problem patients in the first place. One reason, and a simple one, is that the nurse may expect more of herself than is humanly possible to deliver, with the result that she accomplishes less than she is capable of. Let me explain:

One can safely say that most people who choose nursing as their career have a genuine desire to serve mankind and to help those who are in need of help. Yet many young people who want to be nurses have no realistic idea of what "helping" consists of; they usually decide on their career at an early age (1), in high school, when fantasies about one's future accomplishments are still considerably unmarred by facts. Thus, they may see themselves moving blissfully through the wards, dispensing kindness to all and sundry, smoothing out a blanket here, laying a hand on a feverish brow there, always with the result that every patient they come in contact with gives a sigh of relief and enters immediately upon the road to recovery. They see themselves loving every patient dearly as if he were their own father, mother, brother, or child, and finally they see themselves smiling with infinite patience at all times, no matter how

4

numerous their charges, how late the hour, or how sore their feet.

But when these young people enter nursing, they soon find out that often they will be unable to relieve suffering immediately, that they find it difficult even to like, much less love, certain patients, and that there *is* a limit to their patience.

Many a patient may need to suffer in order to get better. There is the patient, for example, who has a fracture and now must put weight on his injured foot; this is bound to be painful for a while, but unless he goes through this pain, he will never be able to walk. Or take a patient who has had abdominal surgery: he is encouraged to breathe deeply and to cough, in spite of the pain it will cause him, in order to prevent respiratory complications.

Then there is the patient who will not get better in spite of the nurse's ministrations. He may have a disease for which as yet no cure has been found; or he may not have the physical or emotional strength needed to pull himself out of his illness. Some patients may even actively fight the nurse's attempts to be of help.

And there will be some patients whose odor or appearance may, at first, be repulsive to any human being. There will be others who, by the way they contracted their illness or by the principles which guide their life (or the apparent lack of them), may stir up an automatic reaction of disapproval in people who have been taught certain morals by their elders. There are patients whose uncontrolled expression of emotions may greatly disquiet others who have, since childhood, practiced self-control.

Finally, the nurse may find that her temper has its variations: it tends to be longer and quite docile after a day away from duty or when she has a reasonable workload and cooperative patients and coworkers; it may have a tendency to become rather short and hard to control toward the end of a day burdened with harassing emergencies, shortage of staff, and patients who seem to have no realization of how busy she is.

Rarely during their pre-service education do nurses get the help they need in this clash of their original, idealistic hopes for their future performance and the actual situation which interferes with these hopes. Few nurses are aided in broadening their initial, youthful idea about the meaning of "helping," in coming to understand that it need not necessarily be synonymous with "cure" nor even with "getting results" but that it also may mean "standing by," "being with," and "being available to" the patient. In other words, there are infinitely more ways in which the nurse can be helpful to her patient than the ones she has anticipated. She is not only helpful to him if she takes away his suffering but also if she sustains him through his physical or emotional pain, if she sticks it out with him while it hurts, or if she makes herself available to him so he can call on her if things get too much to be borne alone.

It is also true that the nurse is rarely helped to understand that she can use her "negative" feelings toward patients (such as fear, disgust, or disapproval) as starting point to explore her own values and the patient's intent. For example, by being helped to accept the fact that she hesitates to touch a patient with syphilis although he is not contagious at the moment, she can learn something about the strong influence her own upbringing (i.e., the moral tenets of her parents, her church, the school and community in which she grew up) has had on her present outlook on life. This knowledge will help her toward a certain objectivity concerning other people's actions and points of view. Again, if she finds herself getting angry at a patient who apparently on purpose keeps falling out of bed in spite of siderails, she may be helped to see that her anger is perhaps what her patient, though unknowingly, has asked for. He may need someone to be angry with him, so that he can find some explanation for his own anger, which mounts every time he looks around and finds he cannot remember why he is in this strange place. If the nurse can learn to be sensitive to the anger aroused in her instead of trying to hide it from herself (as an inappropriate emotion for a nurse to have), she has taken the first step toward helping the patient to find the reason for his own anger.

Finally, pre-service education rarely helps nurses come to grips with the fact that they are human too—capable of just so much work and stress at any given period, depending on their own ups and downs. Although patience is undoubtedly a desirable virtue for a nurse, she will be of less danger to her patients, and her self-esteem, if she learns about the factors that limit her angelic qualities instead of pretending that she is an angel and then finding that she or someone or something has suddenly cut her wings.

For instance, some nurses who are most comfortable if they have a great deal of work to do may find themselves bored and irritable when the load gets lighter. Others who are used to giving thorough, deliberate care to patients may become quite upset if they are suddenly confronted with a double assignment. In these situations, instead of finding ever new sources of satisfaction in striving toward and reaching increasingly difficult accomplishments, the nurse practitioner frequently finds herself caught up in the unpleasantness of *frustration*.

What is frustration? It is a state of being which happens when a goal is set and the person moves toward the goal but encounters a barrier which prevents her from achieving it. The satisfying feeling of direction and striving gets converted into the unsatisfying feeling of anger, of wanting to hit out. In the comparison we have made, the goal is wanting to be an angel of mercy who relieves all suffering, who cures all patients, who likes all patients, and who can cope with all situations. The nurse moves toward her goal by learning her profession, by taking on a position, and by starting out on a service. The barriers: sometimes the nurse has to inflict pain instead of relieving it; sometimes the patient cannot or will not get better in spite of all the nurse can possibly do; sometimes the nurse finds that she has strong feelings of aversion toward certain patients; finally, the ward situation or her personal condition may be such that it keeps the nurse from giving the thorough, expert care she has been taught to give and wishes to give.

What happens when frustration develops? Instead of focusing on the goal the person concentrates on the barrier—and tries to knock it down, as it were. A nurse may find herself very angry at the patients who bar her from attaining her goal and may attempt to coerce them into cooperation. Or she may blame the hospital for not letting her function as she would like to: it is "they" (whoever "they" may be) who are at fault. Sometimes she puts the blame on herself, upbraids herself for not being able to help her patients, for being inadequate and incompetent. Carried to extremes, every one of these reactions may prove harmful to the patient *and* to the nurse. She may be pushing a patient too hard; she may feel so victimized by the hospital authorities that her picture of the world may become seriously distorted; or she may become overwhelmed to a degree of complete incapacitation by her feelings of inadequacy and helplessness. In some nurses the feelings of anger may not be expressed openly, but will be kept back in the body, as it were. As a result the nurse will find herself feeling very tired; she will need extra sleep and may have to skip a day of work here and there to get over her extreme feeling of fatigue. As a result, she may wake up some day to discover that she has lost her job.

None of these reactions solve the real situation; for, unfortunately, the barriers have become more real than the original goals. And then it happens that the nurse, finding herself repeatedly barred from what she had hoped to do and be, becomes quite discouraged after a while. She will be disillusioned perhaps, or she will just stop caring; some-

times she may even become cynical. In Part III of this book
I shall attempt to show ways of coping with frustrations
without necessarily blaming the patients, the administration,
or oneself—and without getting disillusioned.

SUGGESTED READING

Newer Dimensions of Patient Care by Esther Lucile Brown
(Russell Sage Foundation: Vol. I, 1961; Vol. II, 1962; Vol. III,
1963).
This gives a very good description of what the hospital situation is like and what nurses' problems are.

Chapter 2
The Nurse May Wish to Please Everybody

There is nothing wrong with wanting to be liked by others and wishing to please. It becomes a problem only if the need to please interferes with one's better judgment and thus reduces effective functioning.

Naturally, many nurses want not only to be good nurses in their own eyes but also want their patients to think so. But to many people the good nurse is the one who responds to *their* whims and wishes, without regard for the needs of any other patients.

Let us suppose that five patients ring the bell at the same time and each one wants something from the nurse. One wants his dressing changed, one wants fresh ice water, one wants a bedpan, the next one is cold and wants a blanket, and the fifth wants the nurse to get in touch with his doctor immediately. Of course, the nurse has learned to distinguish what is more and what is less important and to meet the most important needs first. What she frequently has not learned is to reconcile her innate desire to please and serve to the utmost (and at the same time to be appreciated for what she does) with the necessary setting of reasonable limits, for everyone's good. So, since she likes all her patients and would like them all to be satisfied with her service, the nurse may find herself turning around her own axis, finding it difficult to decide which request to fill first. And then, wouldn't you know it, a sixth bell rings. By now the nurse may be furious: "How do they expect me to help them if they won't give me a chance to do so?"

It is also only natural that the nurse would like to get recognition from her superiors, her head nurse and her supervisors. They will like the nurse, the chances are, if she does her work quietly and efficiently and, especially, quickly; if she finishes on time and is not hanging around when the next shift comes on. On the other hand, she knows that some patients take a long time to get comfortable. Some need a listener, some need extra little things such as a special pillow, or heel supports, or help with their hair. The nurse may feel guilty if she does not take time to do these extras, because it means not doing the good job she knows can be done. Yet she may feel guilty if she "dawdles" with a patient, because that means that she will need help from other nurses to get her work done in time. The head nurse won't like that, and may even make a remark about it to the supervisor. It is understandable, therefore, that the nurse may consider patients who need extra care or make extra demands on her as a threat to her inner peace.

A nurse usually also wants to be liked by her coworkers—another reason for her to do her share of work in the alloted time. To be liked by them, she is expected also to be a nurse of the *same opinion* as the other nurses. For example, if her colleagues consider a patient to be a pest because he smokes in bed, she may have to agree with them rather than show them up in a bad light by her understanding of this patient: Full of anxiety, because of the uncertain nature of his illness, the patient who is a heavy smoker finds it intolerable to increase his already heavy load by cutting out smoking, too. In cases like this the patient is often made responsible for the nurse's quandaries.

Finally, the nurse usually wants to be liked by the physician. This may mean, quite often, that if she is attractive to him, she should not flinch but go along gracefully when he is inclined to pinch one of her various cheeks. It also may mean that she should go along with his orders without questioning his authority, unless, of course, he has made an error in his prescription; then it is her duty to point this out to him. He is, after all, the "boss." Suppose the physician orders oxygen nasally for an old man who is dyspneic. But the old man is also very apprehensive about the outcome of his illness. The nurse knows that getting oxygen means to him that he is not far from death. She cannot reason with him because he is too upset. So she tries to explain to the doctor that the chances are the old man will struggle against the insertion of the catheter, that he will be more upset, hence need more air, and become even more dyspneic. But the doctor becomes annoyed and tells the nurse that doctors, not patients, "give the orders around here." The nurse will have to continue working with this doctor in the future; she needs to get along with him. Hence is it not simpler just to force the patient, or else write "refused" in the chart? And is it not natural that the nurse will feel resentful toward a patient who, as she sees it, has put her on the spot?

What is common to all these examples is that the nurse is *in conflict,* i.e., she is trying to reach two (or more) opposing goals at the same time, and, as a result, is stuck midway between the two: in this instance to be liked by patients, coworkers, and doctors, and at the same time to live up to her own ideal of a good nurse. (Theoretically these goals need not be incompatible, but I think the practitioner knows from experience that they often are.) The nurse begins to move in the direction of the goals: she goes on duty, begins her work, starts to meet demands and deadlines, carries out her doctors' orders. Then she hesitates and vacillates: in which direction is she to go? Five bells at the same time. Instead of answering any one of them, the nurse may stand, as if paralyzed, in her office or find herself running back and forth in the corridor without reaching any of the rooms.

Instead of moving quickly through her work or taking extra time for one patient, the nurse may succumb to the irresistable urge for a cup of coffee, thus postponing her decision. Instead of agreeing or disagreeing with a colleague who berates a patient, the nurse may find herself unable to utter a word. Instead of giving the oxygen *or* calling the doctor back, the nurse may freeze into inaction in front of the telephone. She expends just as much energy by standing still as she would by moving in one direction or another, because she virtually goes in two opposite directions at the same time. Hence nurses may frequently feel very tired, though they have not done a great deal of work.

A person will stop hesitating and vacillating once she is able to make a choice. Several solutions are possible: One can choose one goal and abandon the other; one can abandon both and look for a third; and one can also withdraw from the situation altogether. Of course, in order to be able to make one of these choices (except perhaps for the last one), one needs to be aware that one is in conflict and know what the opposing goals are. In all the situations I have described above, the nurse is probably aware of alternatives of *action,* i.e., which bell to answer first, whether to call the doctor or just give the oxygen in spite of the patient's fears, etc. But unless she gets help with developing appropriate skills, she may not be aware of the fact that she is caught in a conflict, and may not know what her opposing *goals* are.

In our case she is torn between her goal to feel secure (to be liked) and to feel satisfaction (to do a good professional job). By going after security, she will come to dislike herself for not sticking with her professional principles and will eventually thoroughly dislike those people whom she sought to please. On the other hand, she will have to cope with a great deal of discomfort if she consistently sticks to her principles; as a result she may be loathed by everyone she comes in contact with. The decision, if she is aware of all its components and has learned to weigh the facts, will probably be somewhere in the middle. It may lean more heavily in the direction of security if conditions are overwhelming, if the issue is so trivial that it does not warrant a fight, or if the situation is such that she would through possible reprisals endanger the patient by sticking to her guns. It may also lean in the direction of security if she does not feel up to par for personal reasons. Her decision may lean more heavily in the direction of satisfaction if the issue is an important one, if she has some support from at least one person on the staff or the patient and his family, or if she herself feels strong and able to stand alone. This will be easier to do if, in her pre-service education, the nurse has been helped to understand that the meaning of "professional service" has less to do with "servility" and submission than with offering to share with those who need them one's educated knowledge, skills, and attitudes (see Chapter 12). It will be also easier if the nurse is reminded that, in her professional just as in her private life, it may in the long run be more satisfying to be respected than to be liked, especially if the prospect exists that respect will turn into liking on a higher plane, as it were.

But, as I have said, in order to consider all these alternatives, the nurse must have had help to know what conflict is, how to recognize it in herself, what to look for, and how to arrive at solutions.

In the meantime, the chances are that many a nurse will instinctively abandon the struggle, i.e., turn away from both alternatives, by withdrawing emotionally from any involvement with patients or staff. She may go about her work mechanically, without much interest and without any investment of herself. This, too, unfortunately will turn out to be very unsatisfying, for time spent without putting oneself into it is like paying with one's life for nothing in return. In Part III, I shall attempt to arrive at some constructive solutions.

Suggested Reading

Concerning security and satisfaction, see *The Interpersonal Theory of Psychiatry* by Harry Stack Sullivan (Norton, 1953), chapters 3 and 22.

Some of the same ideas are expressed in different terms (deficiency and growth motivation) in *Toward a Psychology of Being* by A. H. Maslow (Van Nostrand, paper back edition, 1961).

Chapter **3**

The Nurse May Have Unrealistic
Expectations of Her Patients

We have stated before that most nurses are highly motivated people whose primary goal is to help others to lead healthier, happier lives. In their individual schools of nursing they have spent years of rigorous training and indoctrination concerning what is good for patients and what is not. Items such as cleanliness, rest, and a balanced diet stand high on the scale of values transmitted to them by their teachers. So does the need to utilize every possible opportunity for teaching health to patients and their families. Another value is that the doctor knows best. He is the expert who puts the sick machinery back in order, hopefully with the guarantee that it will run until the next check-up. The nurse, as the doctor's assistant, does not know as much as he does, but certainly more than the patient about what the patient needs.* Therefore it is only logical to expect the patient to follow the doctor's orders and to follow the hospital routine as carried out by the nurse, without questioning their wisdom and without interfering.

It is to be expected that American-trained nurses will receive in their pre-service education, along with professional precepts, the reinforcement of certain values in the American culture in general. For example, in the American

* This statement does not necessarily reflect the author's opinion.

culture it is the acceptable thing to "keep smiling," no matter what, and to "grin and bear" one's affliction or pain. Similarly, life, youth, and independence are more desirable than death, old age, and dependence.

There may be a few nurses who have been exposed to values other than those listed, either by virtue of their origin and upbringing, or by having lived in other countries or having been exposed to other values by readings or discussions. These nurses may have been able to gain a certain perspective about their own outlook; i.e., they will continue to adhere to it if it seems useful for their task, but they recognize that other outlooks on life are possible and, who knows, perhaps just as valid as their own. But I would assume that the majority of nurses have no reason to doubt the universal validity of what they have learned in "training" and that they expect their patients to go along with them for their own good.

But what happens to the nurse if a patient prefers to die rather than to get well, or if he flagrantly disobeys the doctor's dietary prescriptions? Or if patients, instead of silently gritting their teeth until she asks them whether they have pain, keep ringing the bell and asking for narcotics? And what happens to her if patients, instead of wanting to get up, so that they can go home sooner, cling with all their might to the safety of their beds?

The nurse responds to her patients' attitudes and behavior like anybody else who expects one thing and finds that something else is happening instead; she responds like anyone else who suddenly finds his authority challenged; in short, she responds with *anxiety* (1).

Anxiety is a sensation inside oneself which indicates that something is not going the way it should be going, that there is some kind of unknown danger lurking around the corner, intent on tearing apart one's integrity as a person. Anxiety is a very uncomfortable sensation to have, so uncomfortable, in fact, that in order to preserve one's sense of wholeness, one tends to convert it automatically into something else before one is even quite aware of its existence.

One way of dealing with anxiety is by avoiding it and thus retreating into safety, a "hands-off" policy, as it were. Thus the nurse may regain her comfort by divorcing herself from a patient's behavior and shrugging it off by attaching some kind of label to the patient such as, "well, he is just a difficult or demanding patient," or "he is a chronic complainer—don't pay any attention to him."

Another way of dealing with anxiety so that it will not come into one's awareness is to convert it into anger: "If there is some danger waiting for me, let me fight it before it gets the upper hand." Hence a nurse may understandably be impatient with someone who challenges her cherished sets of values by telling her that he wishes he were dead. She may scold him and tell him firmly that it is silly for anyone to want to die who has so much to live for.

A third way to ward off anxiety, especially if it occurs in the form of a threat to one's authority, is to act like the person who finds himself suddenly prostrate on the floor because a rug has slipped under his feet: he gets up as if nothing had happened and acts doubly dignified. Thus the nurse whose patient will not get out of bed because he is "still too sick," although the doctor has ordered him to do so, may well check her surprise at his defiance with an extra amount of authoritativeness. She may tell him in no uncertain terms that the doctor and she know better when a patient is ready to get up and that he should stop being a sissy.

Finally, one can prevent anxiety from reaching conscious awareness by keeping it tied to one's body. Thus the nurse may suddenly have a headache, or an upset stomach, or her limbs may feel heavy with fatigue. As a result, she will concentrate on her symptom rather than on the anxiety-provoking event. And so, while suddenly feeling very tired, she may stoically remove the neighbors ice cream dish from

the diabetic patient's tray and let him off with a simple "Now you know better than that." Or she may use the intercom to answer the patient who wants to be turned again five minutes after she has made him comfortable: "Look, I have just settled you down, my back is still sore from it, you will just have to wait a little now."

Although all these maneuvers will momentarily reduce the nurse's emotional discomfort and will help her to preserve her sense of integrity, they do nothing for the patient. They also do very little for the nurse in the long run, except for having given her a breathing spell; very soon again she will find herself in a similar predicament.

And the patients, of course, remain problem patients to her, until she can gather the necessary strength and security to let the anxiety come into her awareness without feeling too threatened by it. They will remain problem patients until the nurse feels secure enough to recognize anxiety for what it is, i.e., until she can ask herself whether the patient has perhaps acted differently from the way she had expected him to act, or whether he has seriously challenged her right to be the authority in matters concerning his welfare.

With a great deal of support from others until one has gained sufficient inner security and skill, one can learn to welcome every occurrence of anxiety (instead of avoiding it as a threat) as a challenge to look at what is happening: "What is it the patient says or does to which I react with such sensitivity? What is it that I am so sensitive about?" Questions like this will help the nurse to look at her own values with a new perspective, which in turn will free her to explore those held by the patient. Without some understanding of how the patient sees the world, it is useless for the nurse to try to teach him her point of view, for he too reacts with anxiety when his expectations are not met or when his need to be recognized as an authority in his own right is challenged.

In Part III, I shall discuss further ways in which a nurse can obtain a certain amount of objectivity toward her own values and thus can become aware of and utilize her anxiety for the purpose and satisfaction of developing, through understanding of herself and others, a greater potential for service.

SUGGESTED READING

A classic study on anxiety is *The Meaning of Anxiety* by Rollo May (Ronald Press, 1950).

Chapter 4
The Nurse May Be Caught in a Cultural Lag

Not only has the nurse learned certain values which she expects her patients to share, but she has also, in her pre-service education, learned a certain etiquette (shall we say) of how to communicate to patients about her procedures concerning them. For example, she has learned to explain to patients what she is about to do, but she has also learned not to enlarge upon the purpose of her procedure beyond perhaps mentioning its name or translating it into lay vocabulary.

For instance, if a patient comes into the hospital with a high fever, the nurse is to take and record his temperature, but she is not to tell him how much it is. If necessary, she will give him medications to combat the fever, but she is not permitted to tell him about the nature of the medication, nor its specific use. All she is permitted to tell him is that the medication will "make him feel better."

This used to work fine as long as patients minded their own business and did not read up on medicine in newspapers and magazines. If a patient did show curiosity beyond the explanations he was "entitled" to, the nurse could safely and quickly set him straight; she was not authorized to give him any further information and if he wanted to know more, he would have to ask his doctor.

But times have changed. Patients have been assigned a much more active role in their recovery; and the nurse,

21

instead of merely being the doctor's assistant, is an "integral part of the health team," charged with meeting not only the patient's physical needs but also with helping him to come to grips with his emotions. Instead of doing things *to* and *for* the patient, she is supposed to work *with* him now. But what has been largely forgotten in both her pre-service and in-service education is to provide her with an approach to patients which fits better into this picture than the one she has learned.

And so it comes about that the nurse, using her old precepts for new situations, goes from one dilemma into another, leaving the patient dissatisfied and herself feeling that she has fallen short of the goals set for her. She cannot get away anymore with telling a patient "here is a pill which will make you feel better," for his answer is likely to be that he is allergic to a number of drugs and is not willing to take any medication unless he knows its exact name, composition, dosage, and purpose. What is she to say now? "Your doctor wants you to have it" is certainly not a strong enough argument. Besides, what if he really is allergic to this drug?

Or if she brings in two anticoagulant pills to a patient instead of one, he will worry loudly about his prothrombin time and ask her what has been happening to him. If she tries to close off his questions by telling him that all she knows is that his doctor has ordered two today instead of one, he is liable to think her a fool, but she has certainly not reduced his apprehension.

Besides how does one reduce a patient's apprehension? Well, for one thing by being a "good listener." Does she not know this? She tries, of course, but she has never learned *how* to listen. How can she safeguard herself and the patient from letting him pour out more than both he and she can handle? And suppose he does—what is she to do then? How will she stop the flood without appearing to reject the patient?

She knows that she is supposed to give T.L.C. and re-

assurance, but how does one really reassure? According to
her experience, whenever she has told a patient that everything will be all right, he always seemed to look at her with
pity in his eyes, not so much for himself but for her bound-
less ignorance.

Why does she not ask her superiors or her colleagues?
For one thing, she is probably embarrassed, for after all
she is a registered nurse and the least she should be expected
to know is how to handle everyday occurrences such as
patients' questions. Perhaps she also has a hunch that all the
other nurses including her superiors are pretty much in the
same boat, for otherwise *somebody* would bring up at least
one of the questions that concern her, instead of talking
about days off, ornery patients, or checking whether "everything is all right."

It is not surprising then, that the nurse feels a lack of
direction. What she has learned does not work anymore and
there is no one to show her new ways of dealing with the
situations that come up every moment of the day. And so
she really feels quite *helpless*.

Let us take a look at this. Helplessness seems to me to
be what happens when a person finds that one or more of
his abilities, which heretofore have served him to deal suc-
cessfully with his environment, do not work anymore, either
because the abilities have suddenly disappeared or because
the environment has changed. Imagine, for instance, a
person skiing alone in the mountains, who suddenly twists
an ankle or realizes he has lost his way. The feeling is similar
to that of the nurse who finds that her preparation for
talking with patients is inadequate for what is expected of
her, considering the changed outlook about nursing and the
greater sophistication of patients.

The first reaction to such a partial incapacitation is
probably one of surprise or mild shock (see Chapter 3).
This reaction of surprise is quickly followed by a reaching
out to others with the hope that they will, at least tempo-

rarily, lend one their own abilities to repair or substitute
for the capacity which has been lost. But—there is either no
one around or whoever is there is unable or unwilling
to extend this service. It is at this point that the real feeling
of helplessness sets in. The person feels incapacitated not
only in the area concerned (i.e., having a twisted ankle,
or having difficulties with what to say to patients) but this
feeling of incapacitation spreads over to all *other* areas of
functioning, with the result that the person feels as if
paralyzed, in a trap, alone and abandoned in the face of
overpowering external forces or internal demands. Thus
the skier may be so overcome by what has happened to him
that he may simply stay in the position he found himself
in when he fell, in spite of the excruciating pain this causes
him. And the nurse may find that she covers her ears if she
hears a patient in the next room crying; she cannot move
and at the same time is flooded by terrible feelings of inadequacy and guilt.

Helplessness, like anxiety, is very difficult to tolerate and
to accept. Therefore it is only understandable that a person
will be inclined to seek relief from the feeling itself instead
of using it as an indication that a problem is asking to be
solved. And so a person may aim at undoing in his mind what
has happened to him by berating himself or others for
being responsible for what happened and concentrating on
what migh have happened *if*—.

Thus the skier may tell himself, if only he had listened
to his wife and had stayed home on this day, all this would
never have happened; or if only he had been warned by
someone that this slope had protruding roots, he would
have never twisted his ankle. In somewhat the same way the
nurse who must give a tranquilizer (as a palliative measure)
to a patient who is dying of cancer and who asks her whether
this will cure his illness may wish that she had never entered
nursing in the first place, for she is "just no good in these
situations"; or she may secretly blame the doctor for keep-

ing the truth from the patient and so causing him to ask such painful questions of her.

Another way of attempting to seek relief from an intolerable feeling of helplessness is to go into frantic action without thinking first whether this will lead to a solution of the problem. Thus the skier may exhaust his strength completely by screaming for help until he finds himself not only with a twisted ankle but also without his voice. And the nurse may overwhelm her patient with exhortations that no matter what his doubts, he should follow the doctor's orders, after all the doctor knows what he is doing, he will soon be better, etc.

Or the person may rack his brains to think up a way of getting out of the terrible trap he has fallen into. "If only I could fly" the skier may think, or "if only there was such a thing as telepathy. . . ." And the nurse may spend sleepless nights in trying to think up ways of "saving" a patient who looks terribly depressed, refuses to eat, and discourages any questions about what is bothering him.

Of course, none of these thoughts and actions are useful, except to divert the person from his predicament. The situation continues to exist, and the impending doom has in the meantime come closer. And in a last attempt at relief from the intolerable situation of helplessness, a person may revert to feeling *hopeless*: "What is the use, poor me, I just cannot be helped, I might as well give up." This is of course another dangerous attitude, for it too does not lead to solving the difficulty at hand; it may, in fact, endanger one's life (1). This is the attitude which will induce the skier to settle down in the snow, waiting for death to overtake him. And it is this attitude which will induce a nurse to give up any further attempts to come to grips with her problem of how to communicate with patients. She may relinquish all responsibility concerning this area and just go about her routine tasks mechanically, and with deadened feelings.

An attitude of hopelessness is doubly dangerous because it conditions a person to reject outside help, if it should become available, and makes the task of helping very difficult, if not impossible, for the other person. You have probably heard of skiers or mountain climbers who were found half frozen after a long and perilous search, and who then endangered their rescuers by their defeatist attitude and their resistance to following directions. I know of many a teacher of graduate nurses who attempted to show them a way of improving their communication skills in a complex institutional setting, and who, instead of being of help, ended up by being pulled down by these nurses into the abyss of their hopelessness.

There is, of course, another, more constructive way of coping with helplessness, and that is to deal with the *situation,* rather than with one's own feeling of inadequacy. One can acknowledge the fact that one is incapacitated in one area of functioning, that one is helpless in that direction for the time being, but that, thank goodness, there is nothing wrong with the rest of one's capacities. Hence one can put these other capacities to their full use to see what can be done about the situation. This may mean action in some instances, or it may mean deliberate waiting until a fruitful idea crystallizes.

Thus the skier may remind himself that, though unable to move at the moment, he can withstand the cold for some time if he makes use of the extra clothing he has in his knapsack and takes occasional snacks from the provisions he has brought with him. Instead of exhausting himself by calling until his voice gives out, he can call out at regular intervals. The chances are that by evening the people at the ski hut will miss him and will start to look for him. If, instead of giving up, he uses his energies rationally, i.e., if he keeps his circulation going by moving his arms and the good leg and if he sends spaced calls without exhausting

himself, the chances are that he will survive until help is forthcoming.

And the nurse too can realize that, although she does not know what to *say* to patients, she still has her ability to *think,* to *read,* and to *request* that some remedial action be taken by the institution in the way of in-service education.

We shall come back to helplessness repeatedly throughout the book; also, in Part III I shall attempt to give some suggestions as to how to avoid becoming helpless and what steps can be taken to cope with the inadequacy felt as a result of insufficient preparation for working with present-day patients and assuming new roles toward these patients.

In Part I of *The Nurse and Her Problem Patients* we have discussed possible general reasons why nurses have problem patients in the first place. We also have discussed how, as a result, nurses may be caught in the throes of frustration, conflict, anxiety, and helplessness. It is time now to look at the more specific problems.

Chapter 5
The Patient Who Is Uncooperative

By uncooperative patient we mean that patient who seems to willfully disobey the doctor's orders. He gets up when he is to stay in bed; he eats ice cream when he is on a fat-free diet; he does not take the medications prescribed for him. Every nurse can name similar examples.

How does the nurse react to a patient who will not cooperate? Some nurses may argue with the patient and try to convince him of his wrongdoing. The patient may just shrug his shoulders and persist in his "mischief." Other nurses may ask the patient *why* he is doing what he knows is "bad" for him. This question will not get them far, because it is very rare that a person knows the reasons for his behavior. Only after a person knows all the facts related to his behavior can he deduce a reason; otherwise he can, at best, invent one. Again, other nurses may ignore the patient and simply chart his misdeeds. Let the doctor handle it from there.

Going beyond such outward reactions of a nurse, we will examine next what happens to the nurse when a patient does not "cooperate." First of all he represents a barrier to the goal of the nurse to help him (see Chapter 1). Secondly, he represents a threat to her picture of herself as an authority figure (Chapter 3). The patient, in a way, puts an end to her little world where the doctor is the law and she his executive. With the patient acting up, the nurse is a pall-bearer of dead authority.

Furthermore, the uncooperative patient shows the nurse in a bad light to herself, her coworkers, and her superiors. He makes it clear that she is not such a good nurse; otherwise she would stop his nonsense (see Chapter 2).

The patient's seemingly defiant acts may stir up in the nurse long-forgotten memories of how she too, once, wanted to flout the authority of others, namely her parents. And she may not really care to remember some of the humiliations in body and spirit which she had to undergo while being helped to become a "socialized" human being. And there is the nurse to whom the patient's "rebellion" may represent the moment when her younger brother (or sister) had suddenly freed himself from her iron hand and dared her to use force—a very uncomfortable memory, indeed, of power losing out.

You have noticed that none of these reactions on the part of the nurse have anything to do with what the consequences of the patient's infraction may be to himself. I do not mean to say that no nurse would ever think of the patient's predicament first; I am trying to show that the reasons for one's reactions to another person's behavior are often more closely linked with one's own needs than with the issue at hand. And, I think, only after the nurse has become aware of what the patient's lack of cooperation means to her will she be free to examine what it means to the patient.

In finding out about the patient, the nurse will not ask him directly, "Why do you do this?" Her approach must be more subtle, or she will never arrive at the reason for the patient's behavior. She may begin by asking the patient whether he is aware that the doctor wants him to be at complete bedrest, for instance. Perhaps the patient simply does not know what the doctor has prescribed for him.

Suppose he does know. Instead of flying off the handle about his infraction of the rule, the nurse might say quietly: "You know, the doctor wants you to be resting in bed all

the time and yet you are getting up to go to the bathroom."
This gives the patient an opening to explain his action.
Perhaps the doctor had told him that it was all right to go
to the bathroom. Perhaps the patient has strong inhibitions
against using a bedpan. The nurse may have to consider
what, in the long run, will be more harmful to the patient—
the anxiety and discomfort connected with doing things he
abhors or the muscular effort of getting out of bed—so that
she can discuss her questions about this matter with the
head nurse or the doctor.

Suppose now that it is imperative that the patient stay
in bed. The nurse will find that argument and persuasion
will hardly keep him there. She will have to give the patient
an opportunity to talk, for example, about his inhibition
against using a bedpan. Simple words such as "Tell me
about it" or "What is it?" may start the patient talking. It
does not matter how valid his point may be in the *nurse's*
eyes; what matters is that the point is *real to him.* As he
talks about his embarrassment, the patient will begin to
see it in light of his total situation. Perhaps the nurse has
helped him along by remarking that she has some idea of
what he might feel, "And yet, if you give in to this feeling,
you are taking a chance with your health for weeks to come."
She can let the patient think about it for a while, and may
perhaps suggest that the nursing staff could help reduce
his discomfort by quickly removing the embarrassing re-
ceptacle.

Sometimes lack of cooperation on the part of the patient
has to do with his fear of accepting the reality of the illness.
The patient who tries to get out of bed even though he is
to be at complete bedrest is, in a way, whistling in the dark.
By threatening him with the consequences of his actions,
the nurse frightens him even more and, hence, increases his
need to deny that he is ill. Often an opening remark like
"I wonder what you think about suddenly being confined
to bed after having been such an active person" might give
the patient an opportunity to voice his fears—that it simply

cannot be true that he is as sick as he is, for what would become of his wife and children if he were. Gently, the nurse may inquire about his home circumstances. She may let him tell her about the strengths and weaknesses of his family members. If the situation warrants it, she may suggest a talk with the hospital social worker.

By listening to the patient and gently encouraging him to go on, the nurse is not taking responsibility for the patient's actions or for his family. She merely helps him gather his strength so that he may face his own responsibility to himself and his loved ones. Also, the nurse need not take time out of her heavy schedule, but may listen as she gives the patient his bath or arranges flowers in his room. Sometimes it will take a few such listening periods to come to the heart of the matter. In the meantime the patient will, perhaps, continue to disobey the doctor's rules, but then, she could not have stopped him anyhow; or the nurse may succeed in obtaining a promise from the patient to go along with the rules or orders until they both have looked a bit further into the matter.

Another reason why patients sometimes fail to cooperate is their lack of trust in the doctor's competence. Here is an example. The patient after a gall-bladder operation is encouraged to breathe deeply and to cough up any loose phlegm he may have in his chest or throat, but he absolutely refuses to do so. As a result he is beginning to develop a respiratory infection. The patient's reasoning often is quite simple: "What the doctor asks me to do is dangerous, for it hurts. I can feel that, if I cough, my stitches will open up. Hence the doctor does not know what he is talking about. So, if the doctor doesn't know how to protect me, I will have to protect myself." Again, by not trying to convince at first but trying to understand the patient's side of the story, the nurse will be most helpful. The fear of bursting open is very real to the patient, and the nurse must acknowledge this reality. Only then can she proceed to teach, let us say, about the various layers of the sutures.

She will also need to get across to the patient that the doctor is well aware of the pain, but that the pain is not related to the danger of the situation; that, however, by avoiding pain at the moment, the danger of pneumonia in the future is increasing. The nurse can then make herself available to support the patient physically by holding the site of his incision with him, and emotionally by encouraging him to cough in her presence, by acknowledging his pain, and by rewarding him with praise for his courage in spite of the pain.

In essence what we have said about the nurse and the uncooperative patient falls into the following categories:

First, the nurse will have to get some insight as to whether the patient's lack of cooperation disturbs her mainly because of what it does to *her* or because of the consequences it may have for *him*. Then, she needs to examine more closely her personal reaction to the patient's lack of co-operation. (Does he prevent me from being of help? Does he show me up in a bad light with others? Does he remind me of when I was little and was punished for insubordination? etc.) Every time she can honestly figure out her own reaction, the nurse will have grown a bit and will be less defensive and thus more objective toward the next patient. This growth is not something she can achieve in a few weeks or months; it is a life-long maturing process. Once she has accepted her personal feelings, and thus put them outside her relationship with the patient, the nurse can, by questions which ask for description (i.e., "who," "what," "when," "where," "tell me," "go on") rather than for the cause ("why") of his action, help the patient understand his behavior (see also Chapter 22). By accepting his point of view as valid, she will have a basis from which she and the patient can jointly arrive at more constructive decisions.

SUGGESTED READING

The Nurse and the Mental Patient: A Study in Interpersonal Relations by Morris Schwartz and Emmy Lanning Schockley (Russell Sage Foundation, 1956).

Chapter 6
The Patient Who
Gets too Personal

There is many a patient who seems to be unable to accept the fact that he is the patient, and the nurse is the nurse, and that the relationship between himself and the nurse is limited in time and context by his illness. Such a patient wants more from the relationship; he wants to know the nurse's first name, her home address and telephone number, and, if possible, her assurance that she will meet him on a date after he gets out of the hospital.

Usually this patient is a member of the opposite sex (and that's why we referred to "him"), frequently in an age range corresponding to that of the nurse.* You know how uncomfortable one can be made by such "personal" questions. Are you or are you not to tell the patient about yourself? If you go along with him, he will probably proceed to ask further questions, like "Do you have a boyfriend?" or "How does it feel to give young men a backrub?" So the nurse will find it somewhat uncomfortable to give the patient the physical or emotional care he needs, for their relationship has taken on a different coloring than it had before. After the patient has been discharged, the nurse may find him waiting at her doorstep. And then what is she to do?

Therefore, the only alternative, it seems, is for the nurse to "put the patient in his place," better sooner than later, for eventually she will have to do it anyhow. But what happens

---

* But this need not be exclusively so. The material in this chapter is also applicable to patients who would like to assume a mother role or prospective mother-in-law role toward the nurse.

when she tells him to mind his own business? The patient may feel hurt, and it is not nice to offend one's patients. Or he will call the nurse names, or comment on her prim and stuffy manner, and who wants to appear like that in the eyes of others, especially if these others are young and handsome? Besides, many patients will not be put off by the nurse's rejection but will keep trying until she gives in from sheer exhaustion.

So, in order to get around the problem, many nurses will avoid the source of the problem, i.e., the patient. They may even warn other nurses about him, so that eventually he may find himself entirely under the care of sub-professional help.

What, then, is a solution to the problem? Before I suggest what may be done, I would like to remind the reader of something very simple. If someone asks you a question or makes a demand on you, this does not mean you are obliged to answer the question or meet the demand, but you should let the person know you have heard him. I know that most nursing texts say somewhere that you should meet the patient's needs. But, let us be frank, does this imply that you have to meet *every* need of the patient, or can you draw the line somewhere? There are some needs that will have to be met by you, and probably can only be met by you; there are other needs which the patient may very well have, but they may not have to be met at the moment, and not necessarily by you. Remember, too, that an expressed demand is not the same thing as a felt need. If the patient wants to know where you live, this does not mean he needs to know the address. We can conclude that he needs something, though neither we nor he may know what this something is. You can help him formulate his need; you can also help him accept it for what it is. You may decide to meet the need if this is indicated, or else help the patient tolerate it, until he himself or the appropriate person can meet it. Under no circumstances are you automatically obliged to meet any demand or any need of a person.

For example: Interest in the opposite sex is to many people an indication that all is well with them; if this interest wanes for some reason, a person may feel profoundly threatened. Patients are often very fearful of the outcome of their illness. If they are still able to flirt with the nurses, they make believe to themselves that things may not be as bad as they seem. Suppose the nurse goes along with the patient or rejects his advances; in either instance she is dealing with his overt behavior. His fear is still there, possibly unrecognized by both, and just as powerful as ever. Suppose the nurse asks the patient what he would do if he had her home telephone number. (Here the nurse is neither going along with the patient nor rejecting him, but she has set the stage for exploring the need behind the demand.) If the patient just says that he would call her at home, the nurse might again ask him what purpose this would serve. Perhaps at this point the patient will mumble something about evenings and nights. "What about evenings and nights?" the nurse can say, and the patient may proceed to admit that, at night, he feels frightened and lonely, that he worries what will become of him, of his marriage or engagement; after all, he will be scarred for life. The nurse may then gently explore further what it is he is afraid of. Is it fear of rejection by his loved one? Does he think he is worth less now because of the surgical intervention? She can help him bring out his thoughts and feelings, and thus pave the way for him to accept himself. Then it does not matter, basically, whether others will accept him or not; he will have the strength to cope with the worst.

You see what happened to the simple flirtatious remark. The nurse has been able to use it and give the patient professional service which at this time is more valuable to him than her personal sympathy or a statement about her professional status.

Let us examine another example: Some people become personal because they do not quite know what else to say;

they may be afraid of the other person or they may find it hard to establish contact. Upon the nurse's question of what the information about herself would do for the patient, he might say that it would make the nurse more human in his eyes. The nurse then might ask whether, without having information about her private life, he thinks she does not appear human. She might explore how the patient sees her. As the patient describes her, the nurse will have to remember that his perception of her is colored by his life experiences and is likely to be far from accurate or objective. The patient's account will be easier to take if the nurse herself has a pretty good idea of what she is like and how others see her, in general. As the patient talks he may come out with the information that the last time he saw a nurse she was specialling his dying father. As the nurse encourages him to go on, he may come forth with his conclusion that since he is now having a special nurse, he must be dying himself. The nurse may then simply explain to the patient the instances in which special nurses are required, and she may explore further whether the patient has observed other indications that make him think he is dying, and so forth.

The patient may have other reasons for becoming familiar with the nurse. Perhaps he is afraid she won't pay attention to him unlesss he assures her of her attractiveness to him. Perhaps he is frightened by the inevitable physical closeness between him and her when she carries out her nursing tasks; he hopes that if he makes advances she will be annoyed and stay away from him.

Sometimes flirtatiousness is used to cover up a feeling of helplessness. We know that of all people infants are the most helpless. Merely to survive, they are completely dependent on the person who mothers them. As the infant grows up, he becomes more self-reliant. He still needs to be loved, but he can survive without love. He can gain substitute satisfactions from his activities and accomplishments. Now, when an older person becomes ill and goes to the hospital, he will have to give up some of his activities and satisfactions. He becomes more dependent, hence his need for love and protection will probably increase (see also Chapter 4).

Many adults, however, feel very uncomfortable when they have to be dependent on others, especially those adults who as children went through a great deal of suffering in trying to find satisfaction of their needs for love and protection (see also Chapter 8). Many mothers, through no fault of their own, are not able to give their children what they need, and children soon learn that it is unfair of them to ask their mother for more than she can give. If an adult who had such a mother feels a need for being mothered stirring in him, he will often instinctively fight it, so as not to be plagued by very painful memories. He will, instead, convert his feelings of longing into amorousness which, after all, is considered adult, hence acceptable, behavior.

With such patients the nurse had better tread very carefully. It is not up to her to bring into the patient's awareness matters which, because they are extremely painful, he has had to hide from himself (see also Chapter 21). Instead it is better to check with the patient (just as in the previous chapter) as to the differences in his life since he has become ill. If he starts to concentrate on subjects that indicate his discomfort with dependency (not being able to do things for himself, being at other people's mercy, grumbling about the service he is getting, etc.), the nurse can listen to all his complaints and then ask him to think of and list for her areas in which he is not dependent. As he enumerates these, she may also explore with him areas and ways in which she and others could help him to retain or regain his independence. At this point he will probably have dropped his flirtatiousness and will have developed a relationship to his nurse which is much more useful to him at this time.

Finally, some patients will not accept limits, especially if these are imposed by members of the opposite sex. Basic to this attitude is frequently the patient's need to cut a dangerous authority figure down to his size. This attitude also perhaps indicates a lack of respect for the opposite sex and also for himself. By trying to oust the nurse from her professional role and to put her into that of a "date," the patient may be trying to prove to himself and others that women are no good and very weak indeed. The nurse who sticks to her limits may be the first woman in the patient's life who has done so. By her firmness about not giving out information about herself—in itself a rather insignificant matter—she may induce the patient to revise his entire outlook about mankind and himself; if there is one person he cannot manipulate, there may very well be others who are not despicable either. The world may not be such a terrible place to live in after all.

To summarize: We have seen that "getting too personal" may be a cover-up for many things, such as fear of the outcome and consequences of one's illness, fear that a nurse might be neglectful unless especially wooed, fear of dependency, and, finally, a need to manipulate or to demote an authority figure and to prove that women are no good. A nurse can be of invaluable service to the patient if she neither goes along with his flirtatiousness nor rejects it, but, rather, very carefully explores with the patient what his advances mean to him.

SUGGESTED READING

The Nurse and the Mental Patient by Morris Schwartz and Emmy Lanning Schockley (Russell Sage Foundation, 1956).

Chapter 7
The Patient Whose Illness
Has a Negative Prognosis

Death is a difficult topic to deal with for every human being. Some philosophers say that to cope with the knowledge that one must die eventually is a unique and basic human problem.

We can expect that nurses too find it difficult to cope with the prospect of death in general as well as with dying patients. Not only is the nurse reminded by the dying patient that she too is mortal, but she may relive with each fatally ill patient the grief she experienced each time at the death of one of her loved ones. Furthermore, she may despair over the futility of her vocation, for she sees herself as a member of the healing profession rather than as one who ministers to a hopeless cause (see Chapter 1).

Is it surprising, therefore, that many nurses tend to hide behind an armor of professionalism; that some may vehemently deny the truth to the patient and his family or even themselves; or still others are liable to exhibit anger toward the patient, his doctor, themselves, or even fate? By denying the reality of the situation, some nurses may push themselves (or the patient) beyond the limits of their strength, which can hasten the fatal outcome of the illness. These nurses will probably also have to shut off their sensitivity to any clues the patient may give concerning his need for support or for expression of his fears.

Here is an example of what often happens: A patient, in his thirties, comes from the operating room after an exploratory laparotomy. His abdomen had been opened and closed; that was all. The cancer that was found was inoperable. There were metastases in several organs. The nurse knows that the patient will probably die within the next six months. She knows that he has a wife and two small children. She knows, too, that the patient is entirely unsuspecting. She is overwhelmed with all kinds of thoughts and feelings. (Of course, she must not express them to the patient, and she also rarely has an opportunity to express them to anybody.) She will probably feel pity for the patient and his family. She may feel like raging at the patient's fate and ask herself what he has done to deserve such punishment (for in the Western, i.e., the Judaeo-Christian culture, the concepts of sin and punishment are often closely linked with disease and death). The nurse may feel guilty about the fact that here she is up and about and well, and another human being, perhaps about her age, will soon be dead. She may be afraid that, who knows, the same fate may befall her or one of her loved ones before long; or she may be reminded of a death of cancer that happened in her own family. Of course, she is afraid of betraying any of these thoughts and feelings to the patient. To be sure that she won't, she gets used to hiding them even from herself. As she approaches the patient with brisk cheerfulness and an extra layer of optimism, she becomes a living lie, both to herself and the patient.

Matters get worse after a few days when the patient asks why he cannot get his strength back as he believes he ought to. First, the nurse tries to reassure him with clichés: "Well, it takes time. After all, you have had quite an operation." But she knows that the patient is getting worse, and she knows that the patient knows it. Each time, when he has not been able to retain his food, and she comes in to change the emesis basin, he looks at her, in silence, with reproach. Some nurses will continue their reassuring phrases; others try to minimize their contact with the patient; again others become defensive, tell the patient that he is not eating right, or that he should discuss this symptom with the doctor. The nurse will breathe a sigh of relief, in any event, when the patient finally goes home, and she does not have to face him anymore.

But, worse, a few weeks later he is back; his condition has deteriorated considerably. He does not ask questions anymore. When the nurse mentions the future to him, he merely turns his head to the wall. She cannot help but hope that he soon will lose consciousness so that neither she nor he will have to face the lie that is between them, unspoken.

That time does come. The nurse is the one assigned to stay with the patient until the end. If she is deeply religious, it will be easier for her; the patient's death will mean a passing into a better life. In any event, with every dying patient the nurse witnesses the transition of a living human being into something which, at best, is a former person to her, and, at worst, is now a thing that rapidly decays. And again there is hardly ever anyone she can turn to and talk about her feelings and thoughts. It should not surprise us, therefore, that young nursing students may giggle hysterically when they have to give post-mortem care. Nor should it surprise us that many older nurses go about their business with a grim look on their faces, unwilling to become human with a dying patient, his relatives, or even with themselves.

As far as the public is concerned, nurses have succeeded in conveying the impression of being always unperturbed and even lacking emotion. The remark that "even the nurse cried" at the death of someone's child illustrates this fact.

And yet, considering that nurses often from the age of eighteen have to take responsibility for dying patients, it is quite understandable that by the time they are twenty-five, they have covered themselves with a thick armor to

shield themselves from repeatedly experiencing such overwhelming situations. Unfortunately, rigid substances, including armor, have a way of cracking at inopportune times, and
the nurse with a cracked armor may find herself suddenly
much more vulnerable to the impact of her feelings than the
nurse who is used to letting herself feel fully whatever emotion she may have at any given moment.

The reader will have to consider that one can experience
a great deal of emotion without expressing outwardly what
one feels; on the other hand one can also have a great display
of emotion without really feeling it—often, in fact, so that one
will not have to feel emotion. In our culture it is not good
taste to express one's feelings strongly; people are expected
to control their feelings. This means, really, that they
should not display too much emotion, but it is often misinterpreted as meaning that they should not experience it;
that, in fact, there is something wrong with them if they are
very sad or very angry, or very anxious or even very happy.

As a result of this misunderstanding, which most probably has been inculcated into them from the time they were
little, people will tend either to suppress their feelings
through conscious effort or to get rid of them before they
are even fully aware of them. The latter process is called
repression or dissociation. This act may bring relief at the
moment, but it is rather dangerous in the long run, for the
unacknowledged or dissociated feelings do not really dis-
appear. They are ever present underground, held there by
what is probably a tremendous expenditure of energy; and
under stress or when the person is not looking, as it were, the
repressed feelings have a tendency to break through into
awareness with full force, so that control then becomes very
difficult, if not impossible.

It is, therefore, safer for everyone concerned if the nurse
can experience whatever emotions she might have. This,
paradoxical as it may sound, will enable her to a much
greater degree to control her outward expression, if this

should be indicated, than if she were hiding her feelings from herself.

Let us now get back to the nurse and the patient whose illness has a negative prognosis. Although any nurse will have taken care of a variety of such patients, the basic question she will ask herself remains the same. How is she to cope with the situation so that she will be of maximum comfort to the patient and still preserve herself for professional functioning with him and other patients? I think that the nurse, to be capable of kindness and professional objectivity, will have to attempt to solve her own questions relating to death. She may be able to do so by herself, or perhaps with a person she can confide in, either someone personally close to her or a professional listener. She will have to think about what death means to her personally, her own death and that of her loved ones.

She will have to ask herself: can I accept the fact that I too will die some day? If not, why not? Am I afraid? What am I afraid of? Does the fatally ill patient remind me of the death of a person who was close to me? Did I experience the grief concerning this beloved person fully or did I even then have to control myself for fear that my feelings would overwhelm me or show when they should not? Is it as if with each dying patient these feelings of grief from long ago, which I kept from coming to the surface then, are coming up again and again and threaten to take over? And is this why, perhaps, I tend to become too personal (or too detached) with a dying patient? The nurse will have to think further what her family's attitudes are toward death. Do we talk about it freely or does my family act as if death were a final calamity about which it is better to keep silent? Does death mean to them the beginning of a new life or the end of it all, ever threatening?

The chances are that the nurse will not be able to answer these questions readily. To answer them at all may take months or years of search. Perhaps each time a nurse is assigned to a patient whose illness has a negative prognosis, she can consider this an opportunity to ask herself these questions and, perhaps, get one step closer to the answer.

As the nurse gradually becomes more accepting of her own attitudes toward death, she will find that she has become more sensitive to her patients' needs. She will recognize certain differences deriving from the religion, class, and ethnic background of her patients and their families. Older people frequently accept their impending death much more matter-of-factly than younger people. Catholics are frequently more at peace about death, once they have had their last rites, than patients of other denominations. People from lower social strata may be more accepting of it than people from the upper ones, and Negroes more so than Whites, and Orientals more so than Westerners.

The nurse will find that certain patients want to know the truth, all of it. Others, until the very end, want to cling to the reassurance that they are going to live and get better. Still others are willing to accept that their disease will end in death but want to believe that the end lies in a nebulous future.

Of course, the nurse has no right to tell the patient his diagnosis, or even the prospects for the outcome of his illness; yet she can still help the patient. You will remember from the previous chapter (concerning the patient who became too personal with the nurse) that it is usually much wiser to assess what the patient *really* wants to know when he asks a question than to give a quick answer. If a patient is afraid to acknowledge the nature of his illness, there is no reason why the nurse cannot support him with emphasis on the positive aspects of his present state, e.g., by reminding him that at the moment he does not have pain or that the intravenous fluids have helped reduce the vomiting.

On the other hand, there are patients who may need the nurse as the one person in whom they will confide that they know what the score is. If the nurse has made sure that the patient means what he says, and that he is not merely using bravery as a disguised plea for reassurance, she can quietly let him talk about his thoughts and feelings, without either confirming or denying the prognosis for his disease.

Here are a few illustrations: Suppose a patient has been put into a special room. He may tell the nurse that because of this he knows that his end is near. The nurse can, instead of denying or agreeing, repeat the patient's remark to him, and question whether a special room means necessarily that a patient is dying. She may even suggest a few alternatives, such as that a separate room gives the nursing staff the opportunity to care for a patient at all hours without interfering with the other patients. If the patient eagerly jumps at her explanation and holds on to it, she may stress the fact that at a point when he should require less care he would of course be taken back into the ward. This is not a lie, for miracles do happen once in a while. If on the other hand the patient looks at her squarely and tells her that he just *knows* this is "the end," she may ask him whether he has discussed this knowledge with anyone else—his family or his doctor or his religious advisor. If he says he has, she may ask him whether he wants to talk about it with her. If the patient states that everyone, including himself, has accepted the inevitable, and that arrangements have been made for his family, the nurse may soberly reassure him that she and her colleagues plan to be with him in his difficult time and that they will do everything in their power to spare him unnecessary suffering.

But supposing he tells her that his family and/or his doctor are denying the truth to him. She may then make a statement to the effect that apparently he does not believe them, since now he is asking her. She will need to remind him that it is not up to her to tell him his diagnosis or prognosis, but that she is ready to listen to what is on his mind.

If, during the talk, she becomes reasonably sure that the patient is able to accept his future, she may let him use her as his ally, without saying so in so many words. The knowledge that there is one person with whom he does not need to put up a front may help the patient to keep up the appearances toward his family if that need be. The patient may even get accross to his family that he knows and accepts the truth and that he wishes they would too, so that he may spend his last days together with them, without walls of false hope and pretense.

If the nurse can follow this course of action, i.e., working on clarifying her own outlook concerning death and learning to differentiate between experiencing and showing feelings and, finally, following the patient's lead as to what he needs from her in his final hours, she will find before long that she is not betraying the goals of the healing professions if she takes care of dying patients. On the contrary, she will find satisfaction in having helped a human being through his last hours in the way he needed and was entitled to be helped.

SUGGESTED READING

The Nurse and the Dying Patient by Catherine M. Norris, in *The American Journal of Nursing,* October 1955.

The Psychiatrist and the Dying Patient by Kurt Robert Eissler (International Universities Press, 1955).

Should the Patient Know the Truth edited by Samuel Standard and Helmuth Nathan (Springer, 1955).

Concerning the "armor" for protection from painful experiences: *Character Analysis* by Wilhelm Reich (Orgone Institute Press, 1949).

Chapter 8
The Patient Who
Is Overly Dependent

There are some patients who will not help themselves to get better but who cling to their illness and seem to act more helpless than they really are. These patients may be suffering from a long-term illness, such as arthritis, which, because of the patient's clinging to a state of helplessness and therefore not getting sufficient exercise, becomes prematurely worse. Or they may be patients recovering from an acute illness or surgical intervention who, although making good progress clinically, do not wish to acknowledge this; they keep asking for pain-relieving medications, or claim that they are still incapable of going to the bathroom and so on.

Many nurses find it difficult to work with such a patient. They feel irritated by his unwillingness to make the effort to help himself. Sometimes they may feel helpless themselves to a degree of exhaustion, because the patient defeats every attempt on their part to get him back on his feet (see also Chapter 4). Sometimes they are so provoked that they become outright angry at or contemptuous of the patient. On top of this, since nurses have been taught that it is not right to be angry with a patient, they feel guilty about their attitude. No wonder therefore that the overly dependent patient, just like the patient who gets too personal with the nurse, ofen finds himself exclusively under the care of sub-professional personnel. This way the nurse can at least save face and will not have to feel guilty about having lost her temper.

Why should nurses tend to react so strongly to such a patient? Why should they be upset if a patient prefers to stay sick rather than get well? Is it enough to say that the patient's attitude is challenging the nurse's better knowledge that every individual's aim is to strive toward health? (See Chapter 3.) Or can one dispose of the problem by looking at it as another example of frustration, i.e., that the patient imposes a barrier to the nurse's goal of getting him well? (See Chapter 1)

It would seem that both factors play a part in the nurse's anger. But more than that must be involved. Why, otherwise, would nursing students and nurses on staff duty state again and again that they cannot understand *why* they are so annoyed about these particular patients. The situation does not seem to warrant such a strong emotional response on their part.

It is well known that people react very emotionally to traits or needs in others which they won't allow in themselves, whether they are aware of them or not. For instance, people with a tendency toward overweight may be quite contemptuous of fat people, and people with a leaning toward over-talkativeness may resent other talkers.

Now, what needs or traits in the dependent patient may remind the nurse of similar undesirable qualities in herself? It is obviously the patient's professed helplessness that gets her goat. Does she always get annoyed when she has to work with helpless patients? No, definitely not. She has all the patience in the world when patients are, as she puts it, legitimately helpless, i.e., when they are paralyzed or unconscious or exactly as helpless as the illness requires them to be. She only gets angry when the patient makes non-legitimate demands for help, i.e., when he could do things for himself but is afraid of the discomfort that might be caused by such an effort. Perhaps these non-legitimate dependency needs of the patient remind the nurse of something in herself which she dislikes and does not want to be reminded of.

Some readers may raise an objection here, and tell me that I am on the wrong track and should start all over again. Nurses are known to be strong and independent people; indeed, they often do support their own husbands. If we look into their background, what do we see? We find that even when they were children many of them had to assume the mother role in the family, either by virtue of being the oldest child or because there was no mother, or because the mother was physically or emotionally incapacitated, or simply because the mother had to go out and earn a living so that the family could survive—all perfectly reasonable objections.

Yet these nurses who had to assume adult responsibilities at such an early age may still yearn for protection and permission to lean on others. But it would have been unfair to demand satisfaction of their longings for dependence because of the circumstances. The only way in which they probably saw themselves deserving of mother's love was by not asking to be babied, but rather by showing mother that she could depend on her daughter.

Now the nurse taking care of patients sees herself perhaps in some ways as a very busy mother who takes care of her flock of children. She will, of course, do everything for them that is necessary for their welfare, but she will become very angry indeed if the patients make, as she sees it, unreasonable demands on her. For after all, mother has work to do. And mothers are not there to baby people (otherwise *her* mother would have babied her too).

This explanation will not hold for *all* nurses who are irritated by overly dependent patients. But all nurses can at least ask themselves whether they can recall any precepts, such as "the Lord helps those who help themselves" or others with similar meanings that were emphasized in their formative years and whether these might have conditioned them against their patients' attitudes.

They will probably not find the answer right away, nor will they ever find it if they try too hard to remember. In

his book *The Conquest of Happiness,* Bertrand Russell (1)
suggests that the easiest way to solve a problem is to feed the
question and all the known facts to one's unconscious and
let it do the work (in practice, to pose the questions and
facts to oneself and then forget about them). In due course,
if one has left oneself open to receive it, the answer will pop
into consciousness and one can pick it up and put it to use.

Once the nurse knows why she is so annoyed with the patient, she may also know that, in her own background, a certain attitude toward a certain behavior was necessary and perhaps good, but that this need not be universally so. She can
tell herself that if she were laid up with arthritis, she would
probably do everything in her power to keep her joints
nimble in order to continue to be able to take care of herself
and others. She can also tell herself that her attitudes are not
shared by everybody and that the patient is not she.

If she reminds herself of these differences among people
each time she is ready to show anger at the patient or to
avoid contact with him, she will, after a while, notice that
anger or avoidance on her part occurs less and less frequently,
and that the need for either is becoming less pronounced.
By accepting parts of herself of which she had only been
dimly aware, she has become desensitized to what she considered faults in others (see also Chapter 3).

At this point the nurse will be ready to take the patient
at face value. She will neither have to blame him nor have to
convince him of the wrongness of his attitude. Instead she
will understand that even the sickest adult prefers to be self-
sufficient and feels guilty if he reverts to expressing needs of
former periods in his emotional development (see Chapter
6). If he still does, there must be a powerful reason for it.
Perhaps the circumstances of his adult life are more than he
can handle at the moment, or else certain needs of childhood
which he has not outgrown for one reason or another, though
held in check so far, are now overwhelming his personality,
weakened by his illness. And while taking care of this patient

...se can make herself available to him, so that he can
exp...re why he prefers to be helpless rather than independent at this time.

Before giving a concrete example of how I would see a
nurse go about this, I would like to clarify what I mean by
"being available so the patient can explore. . . ." I do not
mean by this that the nurse should bombard the patient with
questions about himself. Nor do I mean that she should even
expect that he will tell her about himself, for she is only one
of the many people he comes in contact with. After all, there
are many other nurses, his physician, his religious adviser,
his friends, and the members of his family. He may wish to
confide in any one of these people rather than in her. He
may also choose to talk to no one. What the nurse can do
is to be alert, should he wish to use her professional skill and
to be ready for clues to that effect (see also Chapters 21 and
22). It is hard to predict what these clues will be, but the
nurse can probably recognize them if she refrains long
enough from making too much small talk to bridge silences
which may be somewhat uncomfortable to her—and if she
can stop herself from admonishing the patient that he should
be different from what he is at present. The chances are that
these clues will come in the form of apology about or dissatisfaction with his own behavior, or a complaint about his helplessness or the care he is getting, or in the form of questions
about his illness.

Now, let us look at an example: Miss S., a woman of
about forty-five, of Jewish background, suffers from rheuma-
toid arthritis and has already serious deformities of her
fingers and great difficulty in walking. In order to help her
keep the use of her limbs for as long as possible, she is encouraged to bathe herself (in bed), and to spend as much of
the day as possible in the wheelchair. She is scheduled for
physiotherapy both in the mornings and in the afternoons.
But instead of following through with this program, the patient refuses to bathe herself, she resists being put into the

wheelchair, and often cancels her therapy appointments (see Chapter 5).

When the nurses insist that she bathe herself or get out of bed, she breaks into tears, and as a result the nurses may feel as if they were the most heartless creatures on earth (see also Chapter 2). If they leave the washbasin by her bedside, she does not use it and sulks instead and refuses to eat her breakfast, for one does not eat one's breakfast unwashed. If the nurses do go along with her and bathe her, resenting every motion they make for her because they feel they have been manipulated into this, the patient looks at them almost triumphantly as if to say, "You see, I told you I am too sick to take care of myself."

Obviously, none of these approaches work, and, to boot, much valuable nursing time is lost by having to keep going back to the patient's room to assess her progress, coaxing her or scolding her, and having to do the work in the end anyway.

I would suggest that the nurse reverse the picture completely. To begin with, she can tell the patient that she has been assigned to her, she has been given quite a bit of time to take care of her, that there was no rush whatsoever. In fact, she has an hour and a half for the morning care, and thereafter can be with the patient every half hour to see whether she wants something, and before going off duty, she has another hour to give her afternoon care. This may seem like an awful lot of time, but it will prove to be a good investment. In order to do this, the nurse must, of course, have first outlined her plans with her superiors and have secured their permission to go ahead (see Chapter 2).

What happens if the patient suddenly finds someone who offers to meet her need to be dependent, but at the same time treats her very much like an adult, i.e., shares the plans with her and gives her freedom to make use of this support as she wishes within the time limits allotted? I think that the first thing that will happen is that the patient, instead of exhausting her strength in a peripheral battle (as it were, in an almost spastic warding off of attacks coming from the outside i.e., being forced to help herself when she feels so very helpless) will be freed to gather her forces into herself and use them for accumulating inner strength. She will visibly calm down; she will also, possibly, call the nurse an angel of mercy, the only one around who understands her. The nurse must be prepared for this and not act too personally pleased, nor defend herself against such praise (for both of these actions would again be interpreted by the patient as a demand on her to be different). Instead the nurse will calmly proceed by telling the patient that she will bathe her and if there is anything the patient wants her to do differently from the way she is doing, she should say so.

The patient will probably shed a few tears of gratitude and mere relief. Instead of focusing on the crying, the nurse will go quietly about her business. "You know, I have not always been like this," the patient may say after a while (and here is the "clue" I have spoken about previously). The nurse will encourage her to go on, with little remarks such as "yes" "no?" or "you haven't?" just so that the patient will know that she is tuned in and ready to receive more. The patient will probably tell her that, quite to the contrary, she has been a very active person, in fact an athlete—she even won a few tournaments in tennis years ago—"and then this calamity struck me." The nurse may show that she is with the patient by stating that this must be quite an experience for such an active person as she had been. (She is careful not to state what kind of experience, so that the patient herself can express and formulate what the illness meant to her.) The hour and a half is almost up and the nurse gives the patient fair warning (of, say, five or ten minutes) and reminds her of when she will be back.

When she returns the patient may tell her that she has not felt as well in a long time and that she is almost ready to try to get up now and take a ride to the coffee shop. The nurse should not show a great deal of approval here, because this, too, could quickly be interpreted as a demand on her part that the patient mobilize herself. A matter-of-fact "well, just let me know when you want to go, and I'll help you into the chair" will be sufficient. At this point the patient may again go into tirades about the lack of understanding of the rest of the staff. And again the nurse should be careful not to take the praise too personally nor to come to the rescue of her colleagues. An answer is not always necessary when someone expresses his feelings, no matter how strongly.

As the nurse continues to take care of her, the patient may perhaps tell her that the illness started after her mother died. As the nurse indicates that she is listening (i.e., with remarks such as "oh," "yes," or "were you very close to your mother?"), the patient may continue her story and talk about her loss and how forlorn she felt after it, or perhaps she may not. She will probably before long want to venture out a little on her own—wanting to wash her face and the upper part of her body, perhaps on the third day or so of the nurse's visits. She may also want to resume her physiotherapy on the ninth day, shall we say, of the nurse's work with her. After several weeks she may express a desire to see the social worker so that plans can be made for her discharge.

The initial investment of time has paid dividends: instead of having an unhappy, querulous, and exhausting patient who is getting worse "through her own fault," the nurse has a patient who has progressed satisfactorily and is almost ready to go home. The patient has also perhaps gained a beginning insight into the relationship of her illness to her life situation (more about this in Chapters 9 and 15).

Things will not always work so smoothly, of course, and the nurse needs to be alert to her own limitations and the possible necessity for greater expertise than she has to offer.

Let us look briefly at Mrs. B., a twenty-eight year old, light-skinned Negro who has seven children at home. She has had a hysterectomy and should have been on her feet and back home long ago, but she will not get out of bed and she

will not eat. "I am too sick, my stomach hurts, I can't" is all
she has to offer by way of explanation.

Her husband comes faithfully, tries to reassure her that
all is well at home but that they are anxious to have her with
them soon. She only turns her head away from him and cries.
After visiting hours he asks the nurse how his wife is doing
and looks puzzled. "She never acted this way before," he says,
"I don't know what's got into her." The nurse suggests that
he talk this over with the doctor and offers to make an
appointment for him.

After this is done, she goes back to the patient. She tells
her that she has time to stay with her for the next fifteen
minutes and that she will be back later to give her afternoon
care. The patient turns away from her: "Oh, go away, what
do you want from me? Leave me alone." The nurse, respect-
ing the patient's wishes, says she is leaving but will be back
around four for her backrub.

When she returns, she reminds the patient that she is
back. "What do you want again? I do not want any backrub,
I just want to be alone, I am just no good," the patient may
say. Since this patient, too, has given her a clue that she wants
to say more, the nurse gently insists that she turn over and
that perhaps she tell her a little more about what she means
by being "no good." In the meantime she will just put a little
alcohol and powder on her back and straighten out the
sheet.

As she listens to the patient, the nurse becomes quite uncomfortable. The patient's statements seem disjointed, they
do not hang together. With difficulty, from under the sob-
bing, she can identify statements such as "Oh, what's the
use . . . no woman . . . the Virgin Mary is punishing me
. . . everybody hates me; I'm no good, I should be dead. . . ."

Here, instead of a merely "resistant" or "overdependent"
patient, the nurse has come up against someone who is under
serious psychological stress. (Her own discomfort is a response to the patient's intense anxiety.) She informs her

superiors immediately that there is a patient who is in dire
need of expert evaluation and help. Until such help arrives,
the nurse will spend as much time as she can just being *with*
the patient, or at least, keeping her under close surveil-
lance, for the patient's way of seeing herself and life at this
point may well precipitate a flight into suicide.

In this chapter we have attempted to demonstrate that
the nurse needs to come to grips with her own idiosyncracies
about dependence (by checking into her own upbringing
and the role dependency and self-sufficiency have played in
it), and that she needs to differentiate herself from her patient; they are two people with separate backgrounds and outlooks on life. We have further demonstrated how, instead of
pushing the patients into independence, she can make herself
available to them. While she is careful to treat them as
adults, she can support them in their dependency needs until
they have gathered sufficient strength to move ahead or until
more expert help arrives on the scene.

Suggested Reading

The Nurse and the Mental Patient by Morris Schwartz
and Emmy Lanning Schockley (Russell Sage Foundation, 1956).
   Interpersonal Relations in Nursing by Hildegard E. Peplau
(Putnam, 1952).
   Toward a Psychology of Being by A. H. Maslow (Van Nost-
rand, paper back edition, 1961).

Chapter 9
The Patient Who Is Complaining and Demanding — The Long-Term Patient

A patient's ways of complaining (whether it be about personal discomfort, hospital conditions, or the nurses) or of demanding that instant attention and service be given him (according to his whim) are all thoroughly disliked by many nurses. Sometimes a patient will be both complaining *and* demanding; sometimes one patient does the complaining and another the demanding. Usually these qualities are outstanding in patients who have been in the hospital for several weeks, months, or even years, or who repeatedly return to the hospital with exacerbations of the same illness or with a new ailment at each sojourn. Examples are patients with bone and joint disease, cardiovascular disease, asthma, and mental illness.

Typically the situation is this. A nurse reports that Mr. C. certainly had a personality change since he was admitted two months ago with a fractured femur. It is true that he has developed osteomyelitis since, but at first he never complained of pain and never said anything about discomfort related to the traction he was in. Now he keeps calling for pain relievers every few hours, and if the nurse refuses or delays giving them to him, he starts such a commotion on the ward that the other patients too demand that he be medicated, in addition to asking for headache pills for themselves. Besides, Mr. C. will ring the bell every half hour and ask that his position be changed. And when the nurses start rearranging pillows to make him more comfortable, he will yell at them and tell them that they do not know what they are doing.

What is it that angers nurses so much about these patients? At first thought it does not seem to be a crime to ask for relief of pain or to tell the nurse how to move pillows so as to avoid unnecessary discomfort. I think one of the reasons for the nurse's resentment of such patients is that she does not expect to be told what to do by anyone, except by the doctor or supervisor. As we mentioned in Chapter 3, she respects the customary hierarchy of the hospital, and in this hierarchy the patient is last in line—strictly without expertise and knowledge. "What does a lay person know about what he needs and what movements are best for him?" As things are, the nurse expects the patient to take orders from her and not to issue them (see Chapter 3, and also the footnote on page 16).

The nurse's resentment may also have to do, I think, with the role the hospital plays in the patient's illness. Acute illness has relatively little impact on the patient's worth as a person, as felt by him and others. Though a patient at the hospital, at first he still represents the outside community, and so do his visitors. The hospital is just a wayside service station. Everybody scurries around his broken-down machinery, sounding it out for hidden damage and working fast to straighten out obvious impairment so that he can safely get back on the road again. But sometimes the patient has to stay on after the acute stage has passed, either because the repair turns out to be a long-drawn-out process or because his machinery is in such a state that it cannot be trusted anymore to take to the road. Parts of him may prove useful in the future, but as an entity the machinery won't work.

And so a subtle but important change takes place in the relationship between the patient and the hospital. The visitors, frequent and numerous at first, come less and less often or stop coming altogether. Gradually the community at large recedes into insignificance, and the hospital environment becomes the center of his life. The ward he lives in, his meals, the other patients, the nursing staff, and the doctors are at the focus of his attention. But the only link he has ever had with these was his illness. And there is nothing interesting to his illness anymore, neither to the staff nor to him. The damage is known, all he has to do is to wait for nature (aided by the services of the hospital) to take its course, for better or for worse. If he has no particularly disturbing symptoms he is liable to be ignored by the staff, who are giving their attention to those who are more acutely ill.

As you know, one of the hardest things for humans to take is not to be important to other human beings. They want to be loved or at least liked, and if this is impossible, they would rather be hated, i.e., worthy of at least hate and thus at least be *somebody*, than be ignored, i.e., insignificant, unworthy of anything, a nobody.

And so the patient tries to attract the nurse's attention through the only link he has with her, his illness. He will complain of discomfort or demand medication or care and even create new symptoms just so that she shall not forget his existence.

The nurse, of course, senses that he is trying to manipulate her into paying attention to him and resents this. In the power struggle that ensues, the patient clamors and the nurse acts as if she were deaf. In the end both win and both lose at the same time. The patient finally gets what he asked for, but it is given him with such poor grace that he gets little satisfaction out of it, for all he wanted in the first place was a little sympathy and recognition.

And the nurse, though she has succeeded in controlling the situation, by at least making the patient wait until she was good and ready to give him what he asked for, feels a bit ashamed of herself, like someone who has misused the advantage he has over another person. After all, she is able to come and go as she pleases and has the key to the medicine cabinet, while he is tied to his bed, with his leg suspended in mid-air to boot, and is depending on her for relief. In some ways she may feel as if she had hit a defenseless child.

I do not think that anyone *really* enjoys this kind of power over another human being. In fact, it is frightening to find oneself act against one's better ethical judgment and to feel that, because one's opponent is too weak to assert himself, the darker aspects of one's being are threatening to come to the fore and take control of one's actions.

Knowing that there are laws that protect children, the parents are reminded of their children's rights when tempers flare up. Similarly, I think, being aware of patients' rights will help the nurse not to be goaded into misusing the power she has over them by virtue of the situation.

Most of us have had to acquire a certain layer of hostility while we were being socialized by our elders and our peers, which is kept in check by the accepted mode of behavior we have learned and by the danger of retaliation from others who had to acquire similar layers of hostility under *their* conventional behavior (1). Although underneath we may be kindly people indeed, there is a chance that, if suddenly we do not have limits imposed by the other person with whom we are in contact, our hostility may burst into the open; though it is really not meant for the helpless person, it may be discharged upon him. It is therefore better, both for the nurse and the patient, if the nurse deeply concerns herself with the patient's rights as a human being, even if the community has forgotten about him long ago. Such concern will help keep the power struggle between patient and nurse at a minimum.

How can the nurse reinforce her awareness of the patient as an individual with human rights? As we have noted, his illness as a link gets weak once the illness has passed its acute stage. This would be all right if we were sure that the patient is to go home after a few days. But this we can never predict. Many patients, especially those over forty, do become long-term patients, who either stay in the same institution for a long time or are referred to an institution for the chronically ill; even if they are discharged they are liable to return at frequent intervals. It seems reasonable, therefore, that other links must be established right from the start, which keep the patient's worth as a human being and citizen in focus.

This will happen if the nurse makes it a habit right from the start to see every patient not as someone with a disease but as a person who has suddenly or over a period of time reacted to stress in such a way that his disease is the result of it (see also Chapter 15).

Let us go back to Mr. C. Instead of thinking of him as a man with a fractured femur, the nurse may keep in mind that he is a mason who fell from a scaffold twenty feet high and as a result broke his femur. As she receives him on the ward and makes him comfortable, she makes herself available to listen to him (see previous chapter about "being available"). She may mention to him that this must have been quite a fall. The patient is probably too dazed to say much at this point, but the nurse can get across to him that she is willing to listen to him, whenever he is ready to talk about it. (I have noticed over and over again that there is no one who encourages patients to talk about their frightening experiences. The staff focuses on the physical pathology, and the family are usually so happy that the patient is alive that they do not want him to remember the horrible event or remind them of it. As a result the patient keeps it in his system, and tries over and over again to purge himself from it in the nightmares of his dreams—in vain.)

The next day as she gives the patient his bath, the nurse may again open up by suggesting that this fall must have been quite an experience to him. (You notice that I do not specify or describe the experience; the nurse does not know *what* exactly has happened, and for all she knows he may have hurled himself down on purpose. If she had said, "that it was an awful experience" or something like this, it would be doubly hard for the patient to admit why he really fell.) Suppose the patient says something like "I do not know how it happened—suddenly I lost my footing." The nurse may then gradually explore further, always alert to whether the patient is comfortable enough to continue this conversation. If she finds that it is hard for him to talk or if he starts to perspire or if he changes the subject, the nurse can be reasonably sure that he is rather anxious and therefore she had better tread carefully. She may suggest that perhaps he will feel like talking about it another time, but that it will be worth while for him in the long run to know what happened so that he can, hopefully, prevent the recurrence of such an accident. And as she quietly continues to bathe him, the patient may start in again on his own: "You know, I was not feeling good that morning, I did not want to go to work." The nurse encourages him to go on. "Well, we had a little argument at home, before I left, on account of my son. . . ." (He tells her about the argument.) "And you were still upset when you got to work?" says the nurse. "I guess so." (She asks him to describe what it was like.) "When you're upset," the nurse explains, "you may see less than usual, just not notice things, and before you know it, there may be an accident."

"Yes, that's true," says the patient, "I remember another time, oh, many years ago, the boy was just a little kid then, the doctor said he must have an operation. I was kind of scared, you know, and thinking about it all day, and before I knew what happened, I was hanging from the scaffold, my ankle twisted. . . . So my wife had to visit him *and* me in the hospital."

The nurse asks the patient to think of other occasions when he felt anxious and something happened to him and what he usually does when he gets upset like this. She suggests that he and she talk about it the next day while she gives him his bath. The patient looks somewhat puzzled and at the same time pleased: "Gee, I never thought this had anything to do with *me*. I thought accidents just happened." The nurse promises him that they will talk about not only why many accidents happen, but that together they will try and see whether, perhaps, they can figure out ways to reduce anxiety which he can use in addition to his habitual ones, so that he will not add to the already existing dangers in his work. The patient is delighted. In some ways it has been worthwhile to have become sick, even if it means economic difficulties and discomfort over a long time. He is learning something which will be useful to him for the rest of his life. He also feels that the nurse is interested in him as a human being and not just as a case.

In practice it may take weeks or months to make the connections we have shown here, but the process will be the same. Each time the nurse gives him his bath or spends fifteen minutes with him during the early afternoon lull, they make a little headway in their discussion. If a patient is approached in this way from the beginning, he will not need to demand special attentions later on. And a nurse, seeing a patient from the human perspective rather than from a disease-oriented one, will not find herself in a power struggle with the patient later on. If a patient comes in as transfer and the damage has already been done, there is no reason why the nurse cannot attempt to undo this damage. She can ask about his life before he was ill and about the changes the illness has brought to his life; and before long this demanding and grouchy patient with "nothing interesting the matter with him" will be seen again as a human being who reacts to his life situation. The nurse will feel satisfaction in having been instrumental in helping another person to know himself better, which in some cases (as with Mr. C.) may save his life in the future. Thus a prolonged illness instead of turning into a degrading nuisance can become a source of growth for both patient and nurse.

SUGGESTED READING

The power struggle is depicted (somewhat gruesomely) in the novel *One Flew Over the Cuckoo's Nest* by Ken Kesey (Viking, 1962).

Chapter **10**
**The Patient Who
Is Incontinent**

Nurses realize that part of their work consists of taking care and cleaning up patients who are incontinent of excreta either through their natural or through artificial orifices. This aspect of their work does not bother many nurses, but quite a few do find it difficult to work with such patients, and that is why I have included this chapter in my book.

It would be all right if the nurse who has this difficulty could stop there and accept the fact that one need not necessarily love everything about one's chosen vocation. I doubt that farmers are enthusiastic about having to clean stables; they take it as part of their job. Nurses react differently, though, it seems to me. Although, probably, most nurses do not mind cleaning up babies, many nurses do have feelings about changing adults and especially about not "liking" it. Some nurses may delegate this activity to non-professional staff; others may gingerly go about the unpleasant business; again others may scold the patient for having gotten himself into this "mess." Some nurses may wonder seriously whether they have, perhaps, made an error in their choice of profession. Others maintain an attitude of outraged righteousness toward the patient; if he has no consideration for the nurse, he should at least have it for his own skin. They have a point, but they also are shifting the blame to the patient and thus are forestalling any serious doubts they might have about their own shortcomings.

What *is* it about the incontinent adult patient that is so upsetting? I think that here, as in other problem areas, many factors are involved, which we should examine more closely.

First, are excreta of adults more unpleasant than those of babies? I think so. They probably have a more offensive odor, but this is hardly everything. Let us look at incontinence in a broader context.

Babies are permitted not to have sphincter control, but it soon becomes an honorable goal to act as adults do. Conversely, it is shameful not to act one's age, for every culture expects a certain behavior for each age group. It is understandable that the nurse feels inclined to scold the delinquent patient as a mother might scold her three-year-old who does not live up to expectations, and thus makes extra work for her (see also Chapter 8).

We can assume that the deep recesses of many a nurse's memory still harbor painful admonitions by her elders when she as a child had slipped back into not being quite as grown up as she should have been.

Perhaps the nurse can activate these fragments of memory and use them in solving her problem with the patient. When was it that these little mishaps occurred in her own childhood? Or, if she cannot remember, when did they occur with her little brothers and sisters or her own children? My guess would be that little "accidents" happened when new stresses were too much for the child and he or she took temporary refuge in a previous state of development because it had the promise of needed protection and care (see also Chapters 6 and 8). Or they happened as a message connoting envy about the love bestowed on a little newcomer to the family and resentment concerning one's placement into a secondary position. Perhaps the nurse can even remember or deduce the feelings she must have had when, instead of reaching her goal (be it respite from new stresses, like the first days in kindergarten, or recognition

of her protest about being second fiddle in the household),
she was scolded for her "childish" acts. These punishments
deprived her even more of what she needed.

I think that many patients who display lack of sphincter
control are acting from motivation similar to that of the
little girl who wants to be babied for a while before she
resumes again her way on the arduous path toward adult-
hood. Many aged patients who find that they are ignored
as people, and also many of the mentally ill who have been
hospitalized for a long time, almost instinctively know that
one way of getting at least a little attention is to soil oneself,
even if it is at the price of loss of esteem from self and others.
When given an opportunity to find satisfaction appropriate
to their status as adults, these patients will soon give up the
childish habits. For instance, one can take the trouble of
getting them dressed and letting them come in contact with
other people of approximately their own age; or if this is
impossible, instead of saying "How are you, Pop?" one can
spend some time showing genuine interest in them as a
person who has lived a life (see also Chapters 9 and 10).

Besides considering her expectations concerning adult
behavior of patients in the light of what is culturally expected, the nurse will also have to think about some moral
values attributed to excreta in our culture. Ever since the
Victorian era anything connected with the lower part of the
body is not to be mentioned, because of a possible association with that taboo, sexuality. But long before that time
there had been an implication of dirt as far as excreta were
concerned. Perhaps this was based on the empirical knowledge that where there is excrement there is sickness. This
was finally proven medically some seventy-five years ago,
when it was discovered that many diseases are the result
of infection by microorganisms and that these are abundant
in dirt and fecal matter. If the nurse can, to some degree,
accept the fact that she is influenced by this dual heritage
from her profession and her culture while at the same time

concentrating on the chemical and biological connotation of excreta, i.e., that they are the end result of a metabolic process, she may have less hesitation about incontinent patients.

Modern technology also has its impact on the question of the incontinent patient. For example, since wash-and-wear materials have become available, many nurses, instead of sending them out, take care of the laundering of their uniforms themselves. This is cheaper because it does not only save the cost of having them laundered, but it also is less wear and tear on the materials. But since the nurse frequently uses her own bathroom (which is often shared by members of her family) to wash her uniform, it is understandable that she is reluctant to get it soiled by contact with incontinent patients (see also Chapter 16, on the contagious patient).

Finally, I think, there is a relationship between a nurse's status (as seen by herself, her coworkers, and her patients) and the amount of direct patient care she gives, which may determine her attitude toward incontinent patients. As nurses have become fewer and fewer in proportion to patients, and as their administrative duties and today's drug therapies (and the recording of them) require more and more nursing time, many aspects of direct patient care have been delegated to non-professional personnel. Hence, in many hospitals, bathing and changing of patients is more often associated with "lower" levels of service than that of the registered nurse. And, *vice versa, not* to give patient care has for many come to be a symbol of high status in the nursing profession. In fact, there is usually a negative correlation between salary level and amount of patient contact among professional nurses: the more patient contact, the lower the salary. A nurse's abilities may often be put into question if "after all these years" she is "still pushing bedpans." If, within this value system, a nurse is compelled to spend extra time in such intimate contact with a patient, it is understandable that she may feel put upon and resentful.

Perhaps the graduate programs in nursing developed in recent years which prepare expert clinicians, i.e., nursing specialists who are skilled bedside nurses, will in time counteract this trend of connecting a nurse's direct care of patients with an act below her dignity. For these clinicians will require salaries commensurate with their education and clinical skills, which will in turn, hopefully, make clinical nursing respectable again.

Suppose a nurse has learned to face and control her feelings about "symptomatic" incontinence (see Chapter 7). She is aware of the origin of her feelings and can now take the messiest situation in her stride. She neither scolds nor avoids her patient, but instead of focusing on the *symptom* of incontinence helps him to regain his *status* and the outlets to which he is entitled as an adult.

But what about patients who have organic defects, such as patients who are paralyzed from the waist down, or patients who are wearing a colostomy bag? Here the problem is more complex for both the nurse and the patient. Not only has the nurse the task of coping with her own feelings concerning incontinence, she is also concerned with helping the patient to accept his condition and to learn to live with it. And this is not an easy task.

Many of these patients—they too are products of our culture—will tend to regard themselves as entirely unworthy of respect, since they are not functioning as adults in this one area (see Chapter 4). They will tend to belittle themselves, berate themselves, and may even become outright depressed. Sometimes their entire behavior will turn back to more childish ways of behavior: "If I am a child in this area, I might as well be one all the way." But as we have mentioned several times before, this does not work, for adults feel extremely guilty if they do not act their age, and the guilt will increase the depression and so forth.

There is nothing more the nurse wishes to do than to

help the patient to understand this and to help him to *accept* his handicap, so that he can resume his life as a useful and worthy member of his community. And so she encourages the patient with well-meaning phrases and tells him about the other patients who have been able to get back into the swing of things, or even introduces him to these other patients.

This may work with some patients but not with many, I am afraid, for the simple reason that one cannot make the best of things until one has accepted what *is*; and one cannot accept what *is* until one has learned to accept what is *not*—in short, until one has accepted one's *loss*. In order to do this, many people must first live through a series of reactions, called grief reactions. (These grief reactions apply to *any* loss situation, whether it be one's pocketbook, a beloved person, one's job, or an attribute of one's body, or one's health in general. I am sure you have had the experience at some time, to a greater or lesser degree. Try to think back when you or someone you know well, had a loss which meant a great deal to you, and see whether you or the other person experienced emotions similar to the ones I shall describe now for the patient who loses mastery over his excretary organs.)

When the patient finds out what has happened to him, he is likely to go first through a state of *bewilderment;* he feels as if someone had hit him straight between the eyes; everything around him is fuzzy or blurred. Sounds come as if coated in cotton or as if from faraway; his surroundings may be spinning around him. He may feel terribly weak. This phase can also be called the initial shock of recognition or panic, i.e., a state of extreme anxiety because of the sudden, unexpected event (see Chapter 3).

In this stage the patient can hardly hear you, and only with difficulty follow your directions, even if you make them clear and concrete so that they can penetrate his fog. But he is definitely unable to make any inferences from your

statements and he is definitely unable to make new adjust-
ments or to learn. What has happened to him is that his
senses and his entire being have withdrawn from the impact,
so as to escape being mowed down by a head-on collision with
it. This "merciful" aspect of the patient's bewilderment
should be respected by the nurse, at least for some time.
If she tries to force him out of it, she may find that his
personality may become a victim of the impact of his
calamity, which may result in a serious psychotic reaction.

After a while—hours, days, or weeks—the anxiety does
subside a little; this gives the patient an opportunity to
notice what has happened to him. But that does not mean
he can take it yet. On the contrary, he defends himself
violently against the pain of realization, by denying that
the event ever happened. He may scream out or he may
quietly shake his head, and he may say over and over again
that this is impossible—he was well only a few days ago and
this cannot have happened to him, there must be some
mistake somewhere.

It would be foolish to attempt to help the patient to
accept his loss at this stage of his experience. He is still not
ready to hear the nurse. He is too busy warding off the
realization of what has happened to him and his anxiety level
is still too high for him to be able to make connections
between the nurse's statement and his thoughts and feelings.
(In this stage he acts somewhat like the heretics or witches
who were burned at the stake during the Middle Ages. He
feels the fire burning his feet, and he has an inkling what
this means for him, i.e., the suffering that still lies ahead
of him. He jumps from one leg to the other, as if he could
avoid the flames, and he cries "no, NO," as if this would
stop them from their merciless task.)

After this *denial* stage has passed, which again may take
hours, days, and even months or years, the anxiety has come
down again to another level, at which it is possible for the
patient to assess his loss and the damage to him which re-

sulted from it. This stage can be called a state of *anger* or *blame* or *wishful thinking*. It does not mean yet that he can accept his loss, in the true sense of the word. He is now at a stage where (as we described it in relation to helplessness in Chapter 4) he would like to undo, at least by wishful thinking, what has happened to him. So he blames fate for what happened to him, or the doctor who operated on him, or his family who suggested that he go to that doctor. Or he blames himself for having listened to his family, or for having done something terrible that is causing him to be punished in such a way. He may also keep saying that he does not want to be the way he is; that he would rather be dead than this way. Incidentally, the patient usually does not say in so many words what his condition *is*. This is still too painful; he concentrates on what is *not*.

His wanting what he obviously cannot have may remind the nurse of the tantrum of a three-year-old who wants to possess the moon. But she had better not point this out to him, because he cannot help himself. He just is not ready yet to "make the best of things." In fact, I think, it is because of the well-meaning remarks of others who want to be helpful that patients remain anchored in this stage much longer than need be. For in this stage they are more receptive to other people's remarks; the anxiety has subsided sufficiently, so that when others talk to them, the remarks sink in and the patients do make connections. But the connection which they will probably make in this stage is that others disapprove of the way they are deporting themselves and that a demand is put upon them to behave differently. This is of course not yet possible for the patient, otherwise he would do it anyhow.

So the patient not only has to gradually get used to his new condition and its possible meaning for his future, but he has also to ward off people stinging him with their well-meant admonitions to pull himself together. He can use only part of his energy in coping with his loss; the rest goes into defense against his assailants (as he sees them). Hence the nurse will do better if, instead of encouraging the patient to accept his situation, she agrees with him (at each of his tirades) that this a tough nut to crack for him. She may tell him that she wonders whether he is angry about what happened to him; thus she gives him an opportunity to express this anger.

After a series of repeated outbursts of blame, the patient will come to realize all by himself that it is useless (foolish, he will call it) to go on fighting something which cannot be changed. Things are the way they are at the moment, and he had better pick himself up—or whatever is left of him—and start all over again.

It is at this time of beginning acceptance, when he still has the pain of his loss combined with the realization that in spite of it, life is not over yet for him, that he will be most receptive to the nurse's suggestions as how he can learn to live with his handicap and to make the best of things. Now is the time to bring in patients who have learned how and who have done well; now is the time for actual teaching and demonstrations, but not before.

In order, then, to help the patient who has lost bowel or bladder control for organic reasons, you need to assess in what stage of grief he is at the moment. If he is still bewildered from the panic of the initial shock, all you can do is be with him and give him some concrete suggestions to help him in matters of mere survival, such as "take another spoonful of soup," or "turn over now." While he is in the denial stage, you can help with letting him express his emotions, without contradicting him. This will lower his anxiety. In the stage of anger or blame, you can help him to identify his feeling and also show him that it is only natural to feel that way. Finally, when he shows signs of wanting to accept his new condition, you can start teaching him how to live with it most profitably.

I am sure that, as you concentrate on defining for yourself the patient's reaction, you will have forgotten all about
your own feelings concerning incontinence.

SUGGESTED READING

In connection with interpersonal aspects of nursing patients
with cancer, the American Cancer Society (521 West 57th Street,
New York) has a great deal of useful literature available for the
asking.

Symptomatology and Management of Acute Grief, by Erich
Lindemann, in *American Journal of Psychiatry, 101* (September
1944) , pp. 141-48.

Chapter **11**
**The Patient Whose Age
Is Different from or
Similar to That of the Nurse**

There are some patients who, because of their age and the behavior associated with it, may present problems to the nurse. Patients who are much younger or much older may often be incomprehensible to the nurse because of their seemingly absurd behavior. Patients who are of about the same age as she is may present a problem in that the nurse may find it difficult to maintain a professional attitude toward them. She can so well understand what they may be going through; and so she may find herself being either too personal with them or, in order to avoid this, too formal.

Let us examine some typical situations. There is, for instance, an adolescent patient of Latin American origin, with an inflamed scrotum. Instead of lying in bed with an ice bag over the inflamed area, he races through the corridor in a wheelchair, a transistor radio blaring from his pajama pocket. It is past bedtime. The nurse on duty asks him to go to bed and go to sleep instead of disturbing the other patients. He asks for a sleeping pill. The nurse asks him whether he has pain. He says no, but he cannot sleep. The nurse says that this is nonsense, a young boy like him should have no trouble sleeping. He laughs in her face and resumes his noisy journey through the corridors. The nurse feels furious and helpless. She would love to box his ears, she would also love to give his mother a lecture on how to bring up youngsters. She mumbles something about hoodlums and delinquents and then tries to forget about him, after having written a blistering note on his chart (see also Chapter 5).

What happened? The nurse used an authoritarian approach—and got nowhere with this adolescent boy. If she had stopped to think first, she might have remembered from courses she took as a student that in many cultures adolescents, just as two-year-olds, have difficulty in accepting authority. They are involved in the struggle of establishing their own identity as apart from that of others; and they are torn between wanting to be treated as grownups and often still needing to be children. This is also still an age where fear or any sign of apprehension must not be expressed openly, lest one lose face with one's peers. Hence, the more uncomfortable an adolescent is underneath, the more defiant he may be in his outward behavior.

Had the nurse stopped to think about all this, she might have handled the situation in the following way. She takes the boy aside and asks him quietly whether anything is wrong. The boy, still fidgeting perhaps, tells her that he is still waiting to hear from his mother. The nurse checks to find out whether his mother had said that she would come or call. He admits that she said it was not sure, because she might have to go to the hospital with his aunt who expects a baby. The nurse asks whether there is any way he can get in touch with his relatives to find out. He says no, they do not have a phone. And it is too late to call the neighbors. The nurse asks whether he has a dime to call in the morning. He says no. The nurse then suggests that he accept a dime from her, as a loan so that he can call at eight A.M. to find out what is going on.

At this point the boy sighs and relaxes visibly. The nurse then suggests that he go to bed and she will bring him a glass of milk and an ice bag; the ice bag, so his inflammation will subside more quickly, and the milk so that he can go to sleep more easily and the night will be over faster. She promises she will be by his bedside in less than five minutes and asks him to wait for her there.

The nurse keeps her promise; she stays with him until he finishes drinking his milk. She gives him the ice bag and asks him to apply it where it hurts. Then she tucks him in and puts the dime on his night table. "You can return it when you get the money." She reminds him of where the bell is and suggests he call her if he cannot sleep. The boy sleeps soundly through the night.

In this hypothetical situation the nurse remembered what she had learned about personality development and applied it by treating the youngster as an individual who needed to make his own decisions, while at the same time meeting some of his dependency needs without actually babying him (see also Chapter 8). Had she insisted on flaunting her authority over him she would not have gotten anywhere, and he might have kept everyone else awake, besides harming himself and exhausting the nurse.

At the other end of the scale we find the aged patients, whom many nurses find exasperating. Which nurse has not yet run into the old lady with the fractured hip who, as soon as everybody else is asleep, starts to cry for help at the top of her lungs. The nurse rushes in and asks what happened. The patient complains of pain. Her pillows are in disarray and she has somehow managed to slide down to the bottom of the bed even though the nurse had positioned her for the night only a short while ago. The nurse tells the patient that she will prop her up again and that the patient will feel more comfortable then. The old lady protests even more loudly and calls the nurse a criminal and uses other invectives which are so insulting that the only thing left for the nurse to do is to smile. This does not help much, of course, because now the patient breaks out into a long lament of self-pity that everybody is out to kill her and she, poor thing, is completely helpless and at her killers' mercy. The nurse finally summons help and, in spite of the loud shrieks of protest on the patient's part, they succeed in picking her up, lifting, and repositioning her. It is at this point that the patient asks for the bedpan, immediately. While someone runs to get it, the damage has been done; she will have to be changed from top to bottom. The nurse is ready to tear her hair out.

I do not know that I have a remedy for the situation as it actually developed, but I think that, here too, a knowledge of personality development (through old age) may be of preventive value. We know that as people in our society grow older, they are frequently faced with physical and economic dependence. We also know that if they had satisfactory experiences with dependence when they were young, they will not mind it too much later. But many members of our older generation were brought up imbued with precepts that they were to work for a living, that they should not burden anybody else with their personal or economic difficulties and so forth. All their life was spent in working hard in the hope for a better future—if not for themselves, at least for their children.

And now they have reached the future. The money they saved has probably been spent in the first years of their illness. They are left with a Social Security income or perhaps a Welfare check. The chances are that they might end their years in a nursing home, for their children cannot have them in the small city apartment. Many members of our older generation also still have the idea that one goes to a hospital to die, rather than seeing it as a place to get help and recover. No wonder they are terrified and defensive and thus hinder progress rather than let others help them to get better. Finally, many older people find a strange and new environment most confusing. One way of getting rid of confusion is trying to find an explanation for it, no matter how absurd, as long as it eliminates the bewilderment. Explaining procedures does not help much; it only serves

as additional proof to the patient that she has been rail-
roaded into enemy territory.

So what is the nurse to do? The main thing she can
do is to anticipate the confusion and the consequent ideas
of persecution which may be followed by panic. She can and
will have to come to her patient repeatedly before nightfall
and remind her of where she is. She will have to point out
the position of the bell to the patient again and again and
by answering it promptly, prove to her that she is not
abandoned, but that help is available the minute she calls.
This often helps to reassure the patient that there is someone
there to protect her from the evil lurking in this strange environment. In addition the nurse should remember that the
patient is probably afraid of being helpless and dependent
and should therefore be allowed to make as many decisions
for herself as possible.

All the advice I have given so far will be effective only
if the nurse has, as in all problem situations discussed
heretofore, thought through her own attitudes, thoughts,
feelings, and expectations concerning people of certain ages.
She needs to remember what she was like when she was an
adolescent—was she rebellious too? Has she, perhaps, still a
little problem with authority herself, hidden under a veneer
of conformity to hospital regulations? And is the patient
doing something to this painfully acquired veneer? What
does she think about becoming an old lady herself some day?
Does the patient remind her of an aged relative? As with
other problem situations the nurse will either be able to
answer these questions by herself, or she may need a skilled
listener to help her formulate her answers.

Now let us turn to patients who are of the same age as the
nurse. We have discussed in Chapter 6 some of the difficulties
that may ensue if a nurse gets caught up in the patient's
attempt to change the professional relationship into a
social one. And yet, with a patient of the same age it is
very hard to remain professional, especially if the patient's

and the nurse's life experiences have been similar. Suppose that a nurse who had a miscarriage herself is taking care of a patient who is in the same predicament. There is naturally the temptation to tell the patient about one's own experience at that time, one's disappointment and suffering. But by doing so the nurse deprives the patient of the opportunity to express her own feelings, which, possibly, may be quite different. For it could be that the patient is secretly very happy that the child did not come to term, while at the same time feeling guilty about being happy. If the nurse tells her right away that she knows all about a miscarriage and knows exactly how unhappy the patient must be feeling, she only succeeds in making the patient feel more guilty. But if she lets the patient talk first, and it should turn out that the patient really responds quite similarly to her, she can let her know that she has *some* idea what she may be going through, since she has had a similar experience not too long ago.

It is good to be aware of one's own experiences and one's expectations from others, so that one can be more objective and sensitive to the needs of one's patient (see also Chapters 3 and 7). But to demand that the patient feel and act according to one's expectations would be grossly unfair. An illness is not an isolated factor in a person's life; it may have an entirely different meaning to two different people, even though they are of the same age, depending on their cultural and personal background, their present circumstances, and the impact it has had on their goals in life. It is important that the patient come to grips with what his own illness means to *him,* so that, if he *has* to have it, he may at least profit by the experience and may emerge, if possible, as a better and wiser person for it.

Suggested Reading

The Vanishing Adolescent by E. F. Friedenberg (Beacon Press, 1960).

The Adolescent and His World by Irene M. Josselyn (Family Service Association, New York, 1952).

Emotional Problems of Living by O. Spurgeon English and Gerald H. Pearson (Norton, 1955).

Geriatric Nursing by Kathleen Newton (The C. V. Mosby Co., 1950).

Group Work with the Aged by Susan Kubie and Gertrude Landau (International Universities Press, 1953).

Chapter **12**

**The Patient Whose Socio-Economic
Background Is Different from
That of the Nurse**

In this and the next chapter I would like to look with
you at the problems some nurses may have with patients
who are different from them because of their background.
In this chapter I shall talk about problems created by
differences in the socio-economic background; in the next
I shall discuss differences in religion, ethnic origin, and
language.

It happens more frequently than not that people will
look down upon or be critical of others or their customs or
expressions, if these others are different from what they
themselves are accustomed to. Nurses are more tolerant of
differences than many other groups; e.g., they have abolished
segregation in their professional organization quite some
time ago, and they think nothing of giving intimate physical
care to patients with skin color different from their own.
And I often marvel at the equanimity with which Negro
nurses accept their white patients' prejudice against them.
Yet nurses are people too, and do find occasionally that they
may have strong feelings against certain patients because of
the radical differences in the patients' values as compared to
their own.

But why should we shrug off or deny or object to the
ways of those who are different from us? I think one reason

may simply be that we were taught to act that way by our elders and that we have not as yet gotten around to examining their precepts in the light of actual facts. The reason for not having gotten around to it, however, is quite significant and possibly even more decisive than the original influence.

Young children are, as you well know, eager to explore the unknown. They ask a great many questions, they often imperil themselves in their explorative escapades. Yet few children will retain these qualities once they become older. Why is this? I think, for one, that they are being discouraged from asking too many questions, because answering them is too taxing on their elders' energies. I think, also, that the child starting to school discovers that it is somehow dishonorable not to know something, both in the eyes of the teachers and their peers. Hence children learn to pretend that they know all there is to be known about whatever it may be, and they learn to divert attention from what they do not know by shrugging it off with some kind of a cliché or label.

In addition, learning about new things, as one goes to school, becomes frequently a painful process, for subject matter is taught according to the sequence set up by the teacher or the school system instead of following the natural curiosity of the child. It is frequently coupled by the threat that knowing is "to pass" and not knowing is "to fail," rather than serving as a starting point for finding out and letting one's imagination come to play in pursuit of the answer. By the time a student graduates from high school or the school of nursing, learning may have lost all the flavor of pleasurable adventure; instead, it is remembered as a chore of which one is once and for all rid, thank goodness.

Therefore if one works with a patient whose ways seem unfamiliar, it seems so much simpler to ignore or deny the existence of the difference, or to look down upon it, or simply to demand that the patient, while in contact with the nurse, adjust to her ways. And yet by thus preserving her inner peace and equilibrium, the nurse deprives herself of the joy of enriching her life. A great deal of energy is expended in denying or opposing something that exists. Would there be need for much additional energy in attempting to accept or at least explore the differences? I have not measured the various expenditures of energy, but perhaps you can try it both ways.

Think, for instance, of a patient who is a vagrant. He comes to the hospital in a state of extreme physical neglect. He is malnourished, dirty, and beset by all kinds of crawling pests. His breath leaves no doubt of what kind of liquid he has had last. His language, if it is English at all, is usually just as unclean as his body and as picturesque as his clothing when he is admitted. The nurse grants him no more than the physical care he so obviously needs; she avoids getting involved with the person inside the grimy, neglected body. She feels disgusted with the patient, or she feels guilty about feeling disgusted, for she has been brought up by the tenet that she is not here to judge her fellow beings. Finally she feels a sense of futility about the value of her care, for she knows that the patient will return to his previous way of life as soon as he gets out of the hospital. Before long, he will be as badly off if not worse than when he was admitted. To me this nurse is more deprived than the patient, for in his own way he may well accept his own *and* the nurse's way of life and does the best he can with both; that is, he does not challenge either way—all he wants is to be allowed to be what he is.

Now consider another attitude. Instead of discounting the patient as a bad loss or being discouraged about the futility of her services, the nurse can think of the opportunity of enriching her life by coming in contact with this patient— a vagrant. For, if I am not mistaken, the chances that a nurse would socially meet a hobo are rather slim. Now she has the opportunity to learn something from him concerning this group of people and to gain some new insights. Hence, as she scrubs his grubby skin, she tries to minimize her own discomfort by concentrating on her task and making herself available to listen to him, should he wish to talk (see Chapters 8 and 21). The patient may not say much, for he is not only quite exhausted but also, probably, not very articulate. If he does talk about his life he will probably focus on certain aspects of it, leaving out others (such as his drinking, I am sure). But if the nurse listens to his hints and insinuations, she will get some idea of how he spends his days, what his living quarters are like, and in what ways his moral code and values differ from her own. She will get some insight into what loneliness means and what drifting and lack of close ties can do to a person. The patient may see his life as the only possible and acceptable choice for him; or he may dimly feel that he is a failure. In the latter case he may blame everyone else for his lot, including the nurse. As the nurse listens, she will gradually experience a sense of compassion for this patient, instead of feeling disgust, disapproval, or even pity. She will feel respect for him and will understand what *acceptance* really implies: taking another human being at face value, without feeling the need to change him so as to fit him better into one's own frame of reference. Strangely enough, being accepted helps people to summon their own forces and to move toward actualization of their own selves, in whatever direction that may be. (We have touched upon this before; especially in Chapters 8 and 10.)

Now let us turn to a patient who comes from a much higher socio-economic background than most nurses. Let us think, for instance, of an important business executive who, while at a directors' meeting, suffered a heart attack. The floor nurse is taking care of him until a private duty nurse can take over. The patient is most annoyed at having been played such a trick by nature; he is used to being master of his destiny. His wife comes in after his arrival. The nurse wonders whether, if her own husband were suddenly seriously ill, she would have taken the amount of time to get herself quite dressed up, which this lady obviously has done. She also wonders at the cool manner in which the wife seems to talk to her husband. She does not know that good grooming and a certain aloof and sophisticated manner at all times may be part of a certain upbringing and need not imply a lack of warmth.

While the nurse takes the patient's blood pressure and sees that he is as comfortable as possible in his oxygen tent, both the patient and his wife express impatience. Where is their doctor? They want him here now—and not the resident. "Go get him, will you." The nurse tells them that their doctor has left orders and will be in as soon as he can; in the meantime she is to carry out his orders.

Neither the patient nor his wife are satisfied with the answer. They have more questions: "When will the private nurse come? How often will you come in? Where can we find you if we need you?" The nurse points out the bell and tells them either she or one of her colleagues will be in immediately. At this point, the patient nods to his wife and she pulls out some money from her purse to give to the nurse. The nurse is most uncomfortable. "Who do they think I am?" she may ask herself, "I am not their servant."

What this nurse has missed is that people express their mistrust in different ways. Those who are well off may try to bribe the people whom they do not trust. Others, who do not have the money, may resort to flattery or, if the mistrust is very strong, sometimes to invective.

Why are nurses so often considered as servants by their patients, while other professionals, such as social workers and occupational therapists, are never considered as such? I think it has to do with the tradition of nursing. Nurses were serving humanity long before social workers and occupational therapists even existed. The nurses who cared for the sick were mostly women from religious orders or wealthy women who needed to humble themselves out of sheer devotion to their cause or, perhaps, also for a reward in a future life; but they were certainly not expecting status or public recognition.

At the time when all the other service professions began to crop up, the connotations of service had changed to some degree (see also Chapters 1 and 2). Nowadays it means to make one's superior education and training available to one's fellow men so that they can benefit from it if they choose to do so; it no longer has much to do with being their humble servant. It follows that a professional in our society is also rewarded by a remuneration which is more or less in keeping with his educational preparation. Some nurses and especially, their employers, however, still have feelings against equating devotion with money; with a result that in this society where people's worth is considered by many as commensurate with their income, the nurse comes out as a person of lower "worth" than her peers in the other service professions.

There is, of course, another point which has been made by leaders in nursing over and over again ever since the last century, and much more urgently in the past twenty-odd years, but which has not found acceptance as yet among the majority of the nursing practitioners. That is, if one wishes to be regarded as a professional one must meet the criteria worthy of a member of a profession. Some of these criteria (which were originally spelled out by Abraham Flexner for physicians) are: Professions use a well-defined and unique body of knowledge which is on a high level; they enlarge this body of knowledge by contributing to it; and they provide opportunity for their members to keep up with it. Professions entrust the education of their practitioners to institutions of higher learning. Professions function autonomously with regard to formulating professional policies, standards, and activities; and they provide opportunity for economic security of their practitioners (1).

Although nurses wish to be regarded as professionals by

their patients, their peers in the other professions, and the public in general, too many of them are still unable or unwilling (for personal or financial reasons or merely for lack of opportunity) to make an effort to elevate themselves to the point where they can, in light of the criteria we have mentioned, demand to be considered as professionals. As a compromise between being a "servant" to the patient and a "service professional," or because they sense that someone has to give professional service and they feel too poorly equipped to do it themselves, many nurses appear to settle down by serving the other professions.

This may sound harsh, perhaps, but I have over and over again heard nurses tell patients that they were unable to see them because of lack of time; *not* because they were tied up with other patients, but because they had taken upon themselves work which members of other professions had unloaded upon them. In other words, it did not occur to these nurses that it was their responsibility to spell out or stick to the time they needed to offer patients the maximum benefit of their care. Their functions were determined by what was left over from the demands their superiors and other professionals made on them.

Yet, if a nurse does make her professional commitment toward her patients a primary obligation, she may have to endure a great deal of disapproval and loneliness. For this is not the kind of behavior which one is accustomed to finding in nurses. It is a dangerous example to her peers who may not have the courage to act like her, and also to her administrators who have their hands full with the status quo and cannot afford to take a stand as far as she is concerned. And so she may be pressured to conform by her own professional group, through disdain or isolation. If this is more than she can handle (see also Chapter 2), it is only understandable that she will be especially allergic to the idea of being treated as a servant.

Once the nurse is more secure in herself, i.e., in her position as a professional, she will not be so offended. She will, rather, understand that the patient is somewhat upset about his sudden loss of power through his hospitalization, that he is quite suspicious of everybody around him, and that he is, in his accustomed way, attempting to regain a bit of control. Once this is clear to the nurse, it will not be difficult for her to get across to him the reassurance that he so obviously needs, i.e., that this has been a sudden and tough change for him, but he has one of the best doctors there are, a man of invaluable experience, and that, if he can summon enough patience, it will not be long before he is back at the helm of his own affairs.

In this chapter we have talked about some of the socio-economic differences between nurses and patients and some of the reasons why it is so difficult to appreciate them. We have discussed the opportunity these patients offer to the nurse to broaden her knowledge if she accepts and explores the differences rather than rejecting and deploring them. We have also taken a look at the present-day meaning of "service" and its implications for nursing and the nurse herself.

Suggested Reading

Nursing for the Future by Esther Lucille Brown (Russell Sage Foundation, 1948).

Collegiate Education for Nursing by Margaret Bridgman (Russell Sage Foundation, 1953).

Patients, Physicians, and Illness by E. Gartley Jaco, ed. (The Free Press, 1958).

For the history of nursing, see *American Nursing: History and Interpretation* by Mary Roberts (Charles C Thomas, 1956).

Chapter **13**
**The Patient Whose Ethnic,
Religious, or Language Background
Is Different from That of the Nurse**

In the previous chapter we discussed some of the reasons why nurses find it difficult to work with patients who come from a socio-economic background different from their own. Many of these reasons will apply to the difficulties nurses may encounter with patients who belong to a different ethnic group or whose language is different from their own.

But there are additional reasons which make taking care of this group of patients difficult. First, by virtue of habit we may consider our way to be the right way, and hence the only way, the American way, to eat a well-balanced diet, value a person according to his income, bear pain and suffering with fortitude, and smile (see also Chapter 3). Many of us may take it for granted that the white Protestant, at least sixth-generation, American male is entitled to more prestige in this country than anyone else (granted that this value was slightly shaken when John F. Kennedy became President). On the whole, however, the longer a person's family has been in the country, the higher his prestige. The immigrants of yesterday will look down on the immigrants of today in a similar fashion as a sophomore student looks down on a freshman.

Yet it seems to me that few of our nurses can count themselves as belonging to the "elite" Americans. First, most nurses are women, hence they are already one step below the cherished ideal. Second, many nurses come from families that

have not been in this country for more than several genera-
tions. Although we tend to expect our patients to conform
to the "American way of life," it is quite likely that our own
values are a mixture between the "American Dream" and
those of the particular segment of the "Old Country" from
which our families originate. Although undoubtedly some
of us are of Protestant faith, there are many nurses who adhere to the Catholic or Jewish religions. Quite a few of us
have parents who still speak broken English, and some of us
may still speak a language other than English when at home.

Granted, it was difficult for many of us to grow up between two cultures. Perhaps we were ashamed to be different
from what the teacher, ever since nursery school, praised as
the best way of life. Perhaps, also, we were different from
other youngsters; we were not allowed the same privileges as
they were, and we felt ashamed in front of them and resentful of our parents for having put us into such a position.
Many of us want to forget what is painful to us, hence we
resent to be reminded of it through the nature of our patients. Some of us, on the other hand, may tend to see a close
parallel between the patient and members of our family, so
that it becomes hard to be objective toward the patient. We
find that we are likely to be too sympathetic or too vulnerable to the patient's suffering.

In any case, all of us have moved beyond the stage of ado-
lescence, which means that we do not need quite as much
approval of our peers as we did then. Perhaps it is time,
therefore, to try to become objective about our early teach-
ings at school; to acknowledge that they constitute our frame
of reference but to grant that there may be other frames of
reference which may be just as meaningful to those who hold
them as ours is to us. People who do not speak English, or
speak it with an accent, are not necessarily inferior to us,
just as we are not necessarily inferior to them because we do
not speak their language.

On the whole, however, people from other countries tend

to speak several languages, while English-speaking people often only know their own. This is simple enough to understand, since one can go anywhere and be understood in English, but Portuguese or Spanish or Japanese are not as widely known.

Since our upbringing consisted mainly in making us good Americans, we know little about the languages of other people and know almost nothing about their folkways, their literature and art, or their patterns of childrearing. In the last few years, since it is easier and less expensive to travel, many of us had an opportunity to go to Europe or the Orient. But while we are there many of us will tend to stay in English-speaking hotels, where the accommodations are similar to the ones in this country. This is understandable, for it is frightening to stay in an entirely unfamiliar environment and not even to know how to ask for simple directions. We are led around by guides who tell us what to look for, in English naturally, for we do not know the language of the country. When we come back, we try to classify what we have seen in terms of similarities to and differences from what we are used to. Only few of us will have the opportunity to assimilate the other country's points of view, or at least to take cognizance of the values and modes of life of other people.

Of course, some nurses do travel to another country and stay there and work for a time. These nurses will probably get a great deal out of their sojourn. But most of us cannot afford to travel, for various reasons. Yet even we can at least learn one other language, preferably that which occurs most frequently among our foreign-born patients, and we can practice speaking this language with our patients. More often than not we shall find that the patients will be grateful to us for making this effort; they will not laugh at our stumbling attempts to do so. (There are some patients—certain refugees, for instance—who may not wish to converse in their native tongue. I would suggest, therefore, that the nurse obtain the patient's consent before she speaks with him in his own language.) I think that this kind of experience will serve as a reminder to the nurse not to fall into the trap of raising her voice with a patient who speaks only broken English. Even if he does not know the language, he is by no means deaf.

Another way of gaining objectivity to one's own upbringing and an understanding of others is to read books written by people from other cultures, in translation if necessary, and to read books and magazines about these other cultures. This way it will become clearer to the nurse why in some urban Negro groups it is not as shameful to have children out of wedlock as it is among white people. The family structure is different, the father has a different role; it is not he but the woman's mother who holds the family together. If the nurse reads about customs among Orthodox Jews, she will understand why a pious man never looks her straight in the eyes. It is not because he is a devious person, but because it is forbidden him to look at women other than his wife. The nurse will understand that if a Jewish or Italian patient complains, it does not necessarily mean she is suffering badly but rather that she is making sure she will get the attention she needs. In reading about Latin cultures, the nurse will find that the woman, although quite powerful behind the scenes, is much more subservient to her husband than her North American counterpart. Latin men have a much more elaborate code of honor and are much more touchy about it than the males of Anglo-Saxon origin. Any remark that may be interpreted by them as being deprecatory—about their children, let's say—may arouse an immediate counterattack on their part, which may express itself in physical violence.

The nurse can finally learn something about the deep and meaningful philosophy which is part and parcel of the background of many Chinese and Japanese people, a philosophy which helps them accept passively the suffering imposed upon them by their existence—even though they cannot pronounce the English "r."

So, if the nurse continues to broaden her outlook by studying the traditions, literature, and art (and, if she has the money, the countries themselves) of the people she comes in contact with, she will soon find that instead of being annoyed about the differences, she can be of real service to her patients. She will be able to give an irate Puerto Rican father the respect and deference he feels entitled to, and as he calms down, to explain to him what is happening to his child. She will be able to pat the Jewish woman in the oxygen tent gently and tell her that she is pleased about her progress, for now that she can complain, she must surely feel better. She will be able to give the German patient an outline of what he is to expect and will take his attitude of superiority over women less to heart than she might otherwise. She may be better equipped to withstand the charm of her male Irish patients and stick to the hospital rules in spite of her patients' enticements. She will not be shocked if the Frenchwoman, who has a tube in her nose because she has not been able to retain food in days, will nevertheless ask her to help her put on make-up before her husband's visit. She will understand that a Catholic relative may be more concerned about a dying baby being baptized in time than the prospect of its death. She will be less outraged if the families of Italian or Jewish patients slip into the sickroom in much greater numbers than hospital regulations permit. She will know that Old-American or Oriental patients need to be checked especially frequently, for they will never complain and yet may be intensely in need of relief.

By giving you all these stereotypes, I do not mean to say that all Americans, all Chinese, or all Italians are *alike,* nor that all Jews or all Catholics or all Protestants act in the same way. Of course there are individual differences, but there is still a certain cultural framework. That is, a person may either conform to his culture or rebel against it; in either case his behavior will be dictated by the culture. Only the rare person will transcend his culture and become a citizen of the world, but this person too will, by accepting his origin, display some of its characteristic features.

As we have seen, the nurse can look at the patient who is different from her by virtue of his ethnic or religious background as a way to broaden her own horizon. She will gain additional satisfaction by giving the patient the understanding that he needs. Even while she is on her way to learning her patient's language or reading about his culture, her attitude toward him will change from one of expecting him to conform to her into "how can I be of greater service to him."

SUGGESTED READING

Patients, Physicians, and Illness by E. Gartley Jaco, ed. (The Free Press, 1958) .

Culture, Psychiatry, and Human Values, ed. Marvin Opler (The Free Press, 1956).

Culture and Mental Health, ed. Marvin Opler (Macmillan, 1959).

Cultural Components of Pain, by Mark Zborowski, in *Social Perspectives on Behavior,* eds. Herman Stein and Richard Cloward (The Free Press, 1958) .

Chapter **14**
**The Patient Who is a Member
of the Same or an Allied Profession**

There is something about patients who themselves are nurses or doctors which can be most irritating or upsetting to many nurses who have to take care of them. What is it that these doctor or nurse patients do that is so annoying?

Actually, professionals who are patients are likely to act like any other patient; only if they act in one of three particular ways are they apt to be rather upsetting to their nurses. These three ways are: They are unwilling to exchange their professional role for that of a patient; they assume the patient role so completely that they seem to have forgotten about their past as a professional; or they do neither but appear to cloak themselves in the inscrutable attitude of a silent observer.

Let us first consider the patient who will not give up her role as a professional person. She will subtly or bluntly warn the nurses that she too is an R.N., hence able to judge any nursing care given to her. Whenever the nurse is in the process of carrying out a procedure for her, such as making her bed or giving her a medication, the patient will ask her to leave the bedmaking to her and just leave the medicine at the bedside, she will take it later—after all being a nurse herself, she knows what needs to be done. The nurse, especially if she is still young and somewhat inexperienced, may be baffled by this authoritarian attitude of the patient (see also Chapter 4). There is nothing in her orders which says that

the patient is permitted to nurse herself. Yet the patient is
a much more experienced person than she is, and knows what
she is talking about (see also Chapter 2). On the other hand,
if the patient assumes the nurse's role, what is *she* supposed
to do? So, after some hesitation, the young nurse tells the
nurse-patient that she appreciates her offer and that she realizes that she too is a nurse but at the moment she is a patient
and she had better act as one and let her do the nursing.
What ensues, of course, is a power struggle, which can result
in a tug of war. The patient pulls the sheet away from the
nurse and the nurse pulls back from her side. The patient
takes her medication out of the nurse's medicine tray and
puts it on her bedside table and the nurse takes it and puts
it back on the tray, and so on. It is all a most uncomfortable
situation. The nurse finally gives in, in order not to upset
the patient further, yet she has a guilty conscience about what
this might do to the patient. She may complain to the doctor
about it, and the doctor may side with the patient or scold
the nurse for having let the patient get away with it. No
wonder the nurse has feelings about patients who are unwilling to relinquish their professional role.

Some nurses or doctors may react just the opposite way
when they are hospitalized. They carry on as if they had
never read a medical text in their lives, are surprised and
indignant if they suffer pain, and are unwilling to tolerate
the least discomfort. These patients, although they ought to
know better, will ring wildly for the nurse if they see a drop
of old blood on their dressing. Or they may be just as upset
and whiny about a little flatulence, as if they had never before seen this happen to a postoperative patient. The nurse
cannot help but feel a little contempt for a professional who
lets himself go to such an extent. She tries, in vain, to remind
the patient that he need not act this way—after all, he knows
better, he is a physician (or she is a nurse).

But in fact, education seems to have less influence on
behavior in stress situations than we might expect it to, es-

pecially if the stress is more than a person can handle. It is not enough to learn about the existence of stressful situations with resulting anxiety and the havoc these can cause in an individual and society. A person also needs to learn to recognize anxiety when it occurs to him and to know how it *manifests* itself *within* him. Most people react in one or two habitual ways whenever they are under stress; e.g., some will break out in hives, others will lose sleep, others may be unable to stop talking, etc. These symptoms are a mixture of the effect of stress on the person and his attempt to cope with it.

There are rational and irrational ways of coping with stress. The above examples I would call "irrational" for though they attempt to reduce the discomfort of the original stress, they add new discomfort by their own nature. Hives cause itching and increased irritability; loss of sleep creates fatigue and increases anxiety from the fear of not being able to function the next day; overtalkativeness leaves one with the impression that one has made a fool of oneself in front of others and perhaps has revealed more of oneself than may be good in the long run, and this also creates additional uneasiness in oneself.

It helps to learn about "rational," i.e., useful, ways of coping with stress which will not get one (or others) into additional difficulties, and to practice several of these ways until they become second nature to oneself. The result will be that in any given situation there will be at least one way available of reducing one's anxiety.

But let us get back to our patients who are professionals. The third group of nurse or doctor patients we mentioned are those patients who just lie low and watch the nurse's every move without comment, except for a noncommittal "fine, thank you" to the nurse's question as to how they are doing today and a polite "thank you" whenever she does something for them. The nurse naturally feels extremely uncomfortable with these patients—as most people do if they get no clue as to how their comments or approach are received by the other person (see Chapters 6 and 8). She needs some indication coming from the patient that she is on the right track with him and is helping him to feel better. She would even prefer outright disapproval on his part to this ominous silence; at least she would know where she stands. This way she feels that she is being coolly observed and that she will be judged for her actions without having been given the chance to defend herself. Who knows, she may be dismissed tomorrow on the basis of this judgment, and whatever wrong she may have been doing may be serious enough to preclude employment in any other situation. Feeling thus uneasy, the nurse is liable to blunder with procedures which she has heretofore carried out with expert skill. She may drop the needle just before she gives the patient his injection and have to mumble something about having to get another one. She may upset the water pitcher over the patient's bed just after she has changed his bedlinen and now has to start all over again. While all this happens the patient just smiles and looks at her and does not say a word, and the nurse feels increasingly foolish and inadequate. In trying to explain a treatment to her patient, she will have difficulty in deciding whether she should explain it in scientific or lay terms and will probably resort to some unintelligible compromise, while again having the feeling of having blundered miserably.

Now what *can* the nurse do? Perhaps she has been a patient in a hospital herself during her career as a professional nurse. Then, too, she can ask other nurses about their experiences. Perhaps she can reconstruct the emotions she had and those the other nurses had during their hospitalizations. She will find that the stories will vary with the kind and severity of the illness and also with the impact this disruption of the personal and professional life had on the person. The stories will also vary with the amount of preoccupation the professional person had with standards of medical and nursing care before he himself became sick.

Then too, one and the same person may react differently on different occasions. If you were greatly apprehensive about the outcome of tests which might have serious consequences for your future, you may well have pleaded almost childishly for a reassuring word from your nurses. If you knew exactly what you were in for and had perhaps a similar experience before, you may have concentrated on observing the nurse's way of handling you or you may have even told her what to do. If you were still under the influence of an anesthetic and overwhelmed by the urgency of bodily needs, you may well have disregarded any previous learning and have sought the shortest way to gratify your needs, regardless as to whether this action would be unprofitable in the long run or even might endanger your life. In thus thinking about your own or your friend's reactions to hospitalization, you will begin to realize that your professional patient's behavior is not as bizarre as it seemed to you at first.

Instead of merely being disappointed that he does not act the way you expected him to act (see Chapters 3 and 8), you may decide, for example, to make the bed together with the nurse-patient who does not want to give up her professional role. Then you can use this activity as a background for letting her know that you wonder what it may be like for her to be a patient after she has been used to being a nurse for so long (see Chapters 5 and 22). This will give the patient an opening to talk (or not to talk) about her mistrust of the care she is getting.

If she does talk, you can check with her on what care she is expecting and what the difference is between the care she is getting and the care she feels entitled to get. I would not be surprised that, if you squarely faced this issue with your patient (without being defensive about the care you are offering), she might suddenly come up with her *real* reason for not being able to relinquish her professional role. It may well be that she is afraid she will never get well, or that she is afraid she will let herself go and make a fool of herself in front of her peers, the nurses. Then it may be time to assure the patient that to you she is primarily a person and only after that a nurse; if she wishes to talk further with you, you will be glad to listen. If she wishes to talk to someone else, such as her doctor or religious advisor, you will be glad to make the arrangements for her. The patient may continue to talk to you or state her preference for another person, but at any rate she will be assured that no matter what happens to her, she is in good hands when under your care.

Similarly, you may mention to the patient who seems to have forgotten his past as physician that you suppose it is very different to minister to patients from being one oneself. As you broach this subject to him openly, the patient may well tell you he is terribly ashamed about not having more backbone than he has, but he just cannot stand pain—in fact, he had no idea what pain was really like. Perhaps you can help this patient save face by asking him whether this experience might have any implications for his future practice, and what these implications are.

As you see, one patient needed the reassurance that she could be "weak" without losing face as a person, while the other patient needed to be helped to "save face" as a professional. You could not tell beforehand, of course, what each one needed. The only thing you could do, as we have described on many occasions before (see especially Chapters 8, 9, 10, and 11), was to make yourself available in case the patient wanted to talk and to pursue the subtle clues given you by the patient rather than making gross inferences based on your own attitude and expectations.

Now let us go to the patient who acts like a snake watching its prey. If you have a clean conscience about your work, you need not be afraid of mentioning to her that you have noticed her observing you very closely, and you wonder whether she would be willing to share with you the purpose

and the results of her observations. Here again you are dealing directly with what *is,* while at the same time giving the
patient an out should she be unwilling or unprepared to go
along with you.

There is no telling what our patient's answer might be.
Perhaps she was just looking at you to give her eyes a focus
while thinking about entirely different matters. You may
have reminded the patient of the time she was young and
gave bedside care. Perhaps she is really studying what it is
like to be a patient, how patients are affected by nursing procedures, and how she can get this point across to her students
in the future. Perhaps she is only wondering what you may
be thinking. In any case, as soon as your patient answers you,
you will have broken the ice. You will feel less on display
and will, consequently, immediately regain your self-assur-
ance and competence.

In this chapter we have applied some previously stated
modes of reasoning and action to the patient who is a member of the same or an allied profession. We have again demonstrated that misunderstandings arise if the nurse expects
patients to conform to her expectations. It is more useful for
everybody concerned if the nurse can check out with the
patient what the transition from a professional role to a patient role means to him, and if she can make herself available
to the patient should he wish to share his thoughts with her.
We have taken a further look at anxiety, what it can do to a
person's functioning. We have also pointed out that knowing
about anxiety is not enough. We must be sure of how it manifests itself in us, and we must know what and how rational
our habitual modes of coping with it are.

SUGGESTED READING

When Doctors Are Patients by Max Pinner (Norton, 1952).

Chapter **15**
The Patient Whose Symptoms or Illness Are Psychoneurotic or Psychosomatic

There are a considerable number of patients among the general hospital population who receive, after a series of tests, the verdict that there is nothing wrong with them, that they are "merely" high strung. There are many other patients who are told that they are suffering from psychosomatic illnesses, i.e., a physical illness which may be caused or at least aggravated by emotional stress.

You are all familiar with such patients. To the group of psychoneurotic patients belong those who come to the hospital complaining of vague backaches, headaches, or cardiac symptoms for which no pathology can be found. To the group of psychosomatic patients belong those with asthma, peptic ulcer, ulcerative colitis, and, according to many physicians, patients with arthritis. In fact, many physicians nowadays consider most illnesses, including infections (also the common cold) as results of stress of long duration (1, 2, 3, 4).

But the patients do not know this. Hence it is no wonder that both groups of patients may interpret the doctor's statement as meaning it is his impression that they are faking illness in order to "get out" of difficult situations or to gain extra attention. They even see a subtle or not so subtle implication that they are emotionally, hence mentally, unbalanced. As these patients look into the mirror and study their facial expressions, they are convinced that they are not "crazy." In fact few of their friends have such controlled, even-tempered faces as they do. And there is no doubt that they are ill, for otherwise they would not have blood in their stools nor would they have joint pains or a backache or a rash on their fingers which resists all efforts to get it under control. So the patients beg their doctor to look some more, for there must be a tangible reason for their feeling the way they do. There must be some remedy which cures the actual organic symptom forever. If the doctor sticks to his verdict, the patients will go to another physician, who, they hope, will take their illness more seriously and who will prescribe medications to make them feel better, or even operate, to look for the pain causing difficulty.

And when some time later the next symptom appears and the patients are rehospitalized, they will proudly display their operation scars to the personnel to ward off any accusations that they had not been "legitimately ill" (see also Chapters 8 and 9).

It is true that these patients with psychoneurotic and psychosomatic illnesses are often on the blacklist of the hospital staff. They do not like such patients, who, they feel, are malingering and who would be all right if only they stopped complaining and pulled themselves together. After all there is nothing organically wrong with them, or if there is, it is due to psychological reasons. Or, if the patients cannot pull themselves together, they should not be in a general hospital. For its staff is not equipped to deal with such emotional disorders.

Is it true that nurses in the general hospital are not equipped to deal with patients who have emotional difficulties? It is true often that the general hospital cannot offer the precautions necessary for acutely suicidal patients. However, the so-called psychoneurotic or psychosomatic patient is rarely suicidal. If only for the simple reason that the anxiety, which is the driving force in a suicide attempt, is bound up in the physical symptom and thus kept out of the patient's awareness (see also Chapters 3, 14, and 17).

If it is not the potential danger of the patient hurting himself, what else can it be that creates this reluctance of nurses to assume responsibility for care of such patients? I think the sources for this attitude are manifold, and would like to explore them briefly, one by one, starting from the general and coming down to the particular.

In the Western culture, ever since the Renaissance, we have become more and more scientifically oriented in our thinking. We do not believe in a statement or alleged fact unless we can actually prove its existence or at least make predictions based on it. Hence we tend to accept that a patient has pain if we have evidence of injury or pressure on nerve tissue. If we do not have this evidence, we are liable to conclude that the patient only says he has pain but that he does not really have it.

Although psychiatrists and psychologists have been seriously interested in finding relationships between cause and effect (stimulus and response, emotional trauma and subsequent behavior) for roughly the past sixty years (ever since Freud and William James), many of their findings are not as concrete an evidence as is a histological section of nerve tissue. Because the findings are not tangible or visible, they are often considered "illegitimate." I remember a patient whom I took care of some years ago. He complained that he could not swallow his food, i.e., it would stay in his esophagus. X-ray examination revealed nothing. He was a bachelor in his late forties and had many peculiarities, one of which was his need for "consolation pillows." Everybody on the staff considered him a likeable, but neurotic, crank. Years later I heard that he eventually had developed a cancer of the esophagus, and had died. I also heard that the staff felt a little sorry about having treated him in a way as malingerer, because he had been "legitimately ill" after all. What did not occur to them was that this man may have been really ill for years with a functional (i.e., neurotic) illness and that the long-standing functional stress may have resulted in cancer (5, 6).

It seems also to be the consensus that physical illness happens to the patient, while it is the patient who brings about his emotional illness. In other words, it is not considered to be the patient's fault by and large if he is physically ill—if, for example, he has a tumor or pernicious anemia. He has little responsibility in getting over the illness, except, of course, in following the doctor's orders. But this is not so if the illness is considered emotional, neurotic or psychosomatic. In this case, the patient is seen as having the choice of being ill or giving it up, just by changing his outlook on life or by applying a little will power. Although nurses, doctors, and lay people have been exposed to theories of unconscious motivations and unconscious reactions to stress, and although much lip service is given these theories in our literature and art and our daily lives, their implication in relation to illness has not yet sunk in.

I am not denying here the possibility of the existence of a free will but am saying, rather, that various circumstances may affect it and prevent it from operating effectively; and that certain diseases (i.e., the functional or psychosomatic) are often seen as resulting from lack of will power. With other diseases, where the emotional component is disregarded, the concept does not enter. I am saying further that, in consequence, the illness with a recognized emotional component is looked upon frequently from a *moral* point of view, with total emphasis on the patient and partial or total disregard for the symptom. The "legitimate" organic illnesses, with the exception of venereal disease, are frequently seen as objective occurrences which "befall" the patient and where the symptom is the paramount focus of attention and the patient almost coincidental to it.

Nurses may rightly state that they know all this, for they have had an opportunity to learn about emotional illnesses and emotional components of illnesses in their course in psychiatric nursing. It is true that most nurses in this country who graduated in the past fifteen years, and many nurses who graduated before that, have had this opportunity. And yet it has been found that few nurses are able to transfer this knowledge to the general hospital setting (7). In order to understand this phenomenon we shall take a look at the usual psychiatric affiliation.

In most instances it takes place in a state hospital far removed from the home school. If it does take place in the psychiatric wing of the general hospital, there is rarely much inner connection between the two services. The courses are taught by faculty other than the school faculty and, as far as I know, little effort is made in general to connect the two, either before or after the psychiatric affiliation. (There has been a tremendous improvement since the Government integration grants have been given to collegiate schools of nursing; but so far, only a small fraction of all practicing nurses come from collegiate schools of nursing.) For many nurses the psychiatric affiliation was an experience from which they learned a great deal about people and themselves, and perhaps also learned that psychiatric patients are not as "crazy" as they supposed they were. But the students did not learn much about how actually to intervene therapeutically with psychiatric patients, and probably even less about how to transfer what they might have learned to the general hospital setting. It was all right in the psychiatric setting to sit with the patient and talk with him over a game of checkers, but in the general hospital there is no time for such "foolishness" because there is "work" to be done. Little was done to help the nurse realize that, in order to have a constructive talk with a patient, she need not necessarily sit down with him but can talk or listen while making morning rounds or rubbing his back. Although in the psychiatric setting nurses were encouraged to talk with patients, only a minority of students were taught interviewing skills and how to establish a meaningful nurse-patient relationship. All the others, who were in large classes (as many as 100 students per instructor), were, rightly, taught how to avoid such relationships, since the necessary supervision to help them in following through in these relationships could not be given under such circumstances. The students usually were taught to stay away from emotionally charged material—religion, sex, politics; they were taught to divert the patient's attention from himself, lest he spill out material which they might be unable to handle. It is not surprising, therefore, that a majority of nurses want to avoid any subjects that might be of significance to a patient and that they tend to keep conversation limited to somatic symptoms and superficial topics. For they have been brought up to be safe in their work, and any intervention beyond superficial conversation could easily become unsafe unless handled competently. They feel, rightly, that they do not have this competence and prefer to turn to patients who can profit from the technical competences they do have to offer (see also Chapters 4 and 22).

And yet, although she defends herself against these "emotional" patients, the nurse does know that they need her care just as badly as the other patients, if not more so; for they need both emotional and physical support. Not only do they need her care but they are entitled to it. But in that case, the nurse is also entitled to have the necessary skill to give this care. If she has graduated, she will need to put pressure upon the school she came from to give more adequate preparation in this area to her successors. As far as she herself is concerned, since she has not had the previous preparation, through no fault of her own, she is entitled to subsequent instruction on an in-service basis in the areas of interpersonal skills. This is just as necessary as in any other area for which nurses are to take responsibility today but are not sufficiently prepared (such as the care of patients with open heart surgery or patients on hypothermic therapy). (See also Chapters 21 and 22.) If she has any doubts about her right to request such an in-service program she can take a look at the report of the Joint Commission for Mental Health and Mental Illness in which the need for professional personnel, which includes nurses, to work in the area of prevention and treatment of emotional illness is stressed most strongly (8).

Besides in-service education the nurse will need to participate in clinical workshops of her community or her nursing organizations. She will, of course, profit from any good courses in interpersonal relations or allied theoretical subjects given by institutions of higher education.

It will help if the nurse does not only partake of these various opportunities in a passive manner but also prepares herself actively for them, by coming to the sessions with questions formed in her mind. One way of preparing such questions (and, I think, a better way than asking, "What am I supposed to say to a patient with ulcerative colitis?") is to base them on data concerning actual situations between herself and the patient. The nurse should make as many notes as possible; she should jot down point by point what the patient did and said, what she did and said, and what she thought and felt, and what her difficulties and questions were in this particular moment. As she looks at her notes, certain general categories of questions and approaches will perhaps emerge.

By doing this, the nurse will find her in-service programs more stimulating. She will also, through her observations and investigations and her formulation of questions, help to contribute to the rather scant knowledge we have concerning the nursing of patients with psychosomatic and psychoneurotic disorders (see also Chapters 21 and 22). Although we find materials about this topic in psychiatric nursing texts, we have done little as yet to test out these textbook statements. Besides, many of these texts see the nurse as assisting the psychiatrist working with such patients, and the majority of patients in a general hospital are not under the care of psychiatrists but of other physicians who, by virtue of their *own* training, are often more concerned with the organic disease process than with looking for its etiology in the patients' patterns of living. And, traditionally, it is really the nurse who is the one to be most concerned with the patient as a person who is ill (see Chapter 9). Hence it is in her province to participate actively in contributing to the body of knowledge concerning patients who have physical symptoms (with or without organic damage) associated with emotional stress. As she develops more skill in this area, the nurse will feel more comfortable with this group of patients and will receive a great deal of satisfaction in being able to extend her services to them.

In this chapter we have explored some of the misconceptions concerning psychoneurotic and psychosomatic illnesses. We have demonstrated that the nurse, though rightly protesting that she is not adequately prepared to care for these patients, has a responsibility in making up this lack in preparation and of working on the establishment of a body of knowledge concerning the nursing of this group of "emotional" patients.

SUGGESTED READING

Emotions and Bodily Changes by Helen Flanders Dunbar (Columbia University Press, 1954). See also the NOTES to Chapter 15.

Chapter 16
The Patient Whose Illness Is Contagious

In the next two chapters we shall talk about patients who present problems to the nurse because of the nature of their illness, rather than their behavior. In this chapter we shall talk about the nurse's reaction to the illness *per se,* and in the next chapter about the patient's family, who may turn out to be more of a problem to the nurse than the patient himself.

Contagious patients, or patients who are on isolation, find themselves frequently not only under isolation technique but isolated from fellow human beings, including to some degree the nurse. If they are on the ward, they are liable to get only the most perfunctory care. If they are in a special room, they may spend hours on end, alone, while dishes will accumulate and no one may come in to clean them off.

How is this possible in a day and age when infection has to a great extent lost its horror, since it usually can be controlled with drugs before it becomes a rampant epidemic? To add to this paradox, in times of epidemics patients never felt isolated from their nurses; on the contrary, nurses were the people who had the strongest, and sometimes the only, bond with them.

I would like to venture the statement that, partly at least, *because* of the use of antibiotics and other miracle drugs in infections, nurses find it more difficult, i.e., more hazardous and hence more unpleasant, to take care of contagious patients than at a time when all they had to rely on was good nursing care.

Let me explain. Donning cap and gown and mask in a certain way, and removing them in a similarly prescribed way; immersing ones hands in a basin with one-half percent Lysol for a prescribed period of time; brushing one's hands with soap and under running water for an equally prescribed period of time, and, finally, using a towel expertly so as not to recontaminate oneself—all of these procedures proved to be safe rituals from many points of view. First of all, there was an exact convention as to what was contaminated and what was considered clean, and everybody followed this convention—and I mean everybody. All registered nurses were initiated to the same procedure, and only registered nurses (or nursing students) took care of patients who were under isolation; sub-professional personnel was not allowed into the room (as far as I know). The nurses could trust each other; they also knew that their supervisor's or teacher's eye might be turned upon them at any moment, just in case they got any ideas of taking shortcuts themselves. Physicians were watched strictly by the nurse lest they slip up on the procedures; and they went along, I suppose, to please the nurse, or to appease her, or because they too believed in isolation technique.

By thus knowing that precautionary techniques were carried out, the nurse could feel assured that the danger of infection to her and her other patients was minimal. I do not know whether such elaborate rituals were necessary for *all* instances in which they were used. But they certainly helped not only objectively, but also subjectively, as rituals do in general, to allay anxiety concerning unknown or dangerous outside forces. In the subjective respect the nurse's elaborate technique served the same purpose as any ceremonial designed to appease Mother Nature; it was serving the same function (of allaying anxiety) as do the rituals of patients with obsessive-compulsive disorders. This in turn helped the nurse to devote all her energy and attention to the care of her patients, without worrying whether she would become ill, too.

The fact that the nurse had a key role in the recovery of her patient helped to strengthen this attitude on her part. For it was *her nursing care* that could make all the difference whether the patient lived or died. Every little while she would encourage him to take just a sip of fluid, even if it was just a drop, for many drops would add up to the amount of fluid needed to eliminate the toxins from his body. Faithfully she would sponge him with alcohol, again and again, since this and aspirin were the only means of reducing the dangerous fever. Of course she wore gown and mask as she took care of the patient, but in spite of this formidable-looking equipment, the patient felt that the nurse was fighting his fight with him and that she would do all in her power to save him. And after the crisis had passed, patient and nurse would rejoice over the battle won.

This description is an illustration of the common phenomenon that people may lose their fear in times of crisis or disaster and mobilize all their energies to give aid to others. It is the fact that they are *needed* and even *essential* to give this aid which seems to keep them functioning so well in spite of their own involvement or loss.

Besides, in those days, nurses usually lived on the hospital grounds, and if anyone shared their bathroom, it was another nurse. There was little danger that she would carry the infection much beyond the sickroom.

Then came the sulfonamides, penicillin, and the other antibiotic drugs. Many diseases, such as pneumonia and tuberculosis, for instance, can be controlled or cured altogether, others, such as scarlet fever, occur in much milder form and last for a much shorter time. As a result of chemotherapy the nurse's importance in the management and outcome of the patient's illness receded into the background. Her main service to the patient now consists in dispensing medications on time, and to do this one need not be particularly skillful or devoted.

Nurses also now have little to say about the placement of patients on the ward. Since the danger of infecting other patients seems less of a threat ("For even if it should happen," reason those who decide on the placement, "there are miracle drugs which can keep the budding infection in check"), it has become not unusual to put a patient with pneumonia or intestinal infection right on the ward with other patients. They will be put there under *partial* isolation, but even that may not be carefully spelled out. In addition, these semi-isolated patients on the ward are likely to be taken care of by the sub-professional personnel to whom the ward is assigned. Furthermore, many hospital wards do not have sinks in them; it takes quite a bit of inner discipline to leave the ward to wash one's hands each time before approaching the next patient. Can you see what some of the nurses' feelings might be about contagious patients on general hospital wards? But this is not all.

Nurses nowadays rarely live at the hospital residence but rather at home, usually with their families which may include children. As we have mentioned in Chapter 10, they wear wash-and-wear uniforms of synthetic materials which may be laundered in the home after they have come in contact with these infectious, but only partially isolated, patients.

All these examples point to the fact that the nurse has lost, one by one, every single factor (i.e., her control over the situation, her important role with the patient, and the safety of the set-up in general), which before protected her from being afraid (for herself and others) and thus enabled her to devote all her energies and skills to give relief to her patient.

When in addition to what we have already described, patients with *suspected* contagious disease are brought in but are *not* put under any precautions until laboratory tests have confirmed the diagnosis, the nurse may be ready to blow her top. She gets little help from her supervisor, because the supervisor too is often quite powerless when it comes to setting up rules. For, like the nurse, the supervisor has been affected by the changing times in her own way.

She must not act the autocrat of twenty years ago, who breathed down everybody's neck to make sure techniques were carried out faultlessly. Nowadays she must be concerned with "good interpersonal relations," which, in many settings, is equated with pacifying everybody and being popular. We cannot blame her for this, for, again like the nurse, she has her security needs (see Chapter 2). And, although the supervisor does not like the situation either, she gets little support from her director of nursing who has her own problems, one of which is the administrator, who wants to get his institution "out of the red," hence needs every available bed-space filled.

And what about the doctors? I think that they too, trust in the efficacy of medications and have perhaps some doubt as to the necessity of all the paraphernalia previously used. Since many doctors visit only one or two patients in a hospital, and after the visit go out into the fresh air, isolation technique is probably less important for them than for the staff who go from patient to patient. Besides, care of patients is essentially a nursing problem, and doctors have problems of their own.

So, we are back where we started. The nurse has the responsibility, but she does not have the authority that goes with it. No wonder that she may hate the source of all this confusion and danger, the patient. And since she does not know exactly what to consider contaminated and what clean, since there is so little emphasis on technique, she prefers to stay away from the patient altogether.

We can further imagine her uneasiness, if a patient is admitted whose diesase proves resistant to medication, such as certain staphylococcus infections. Now she is back where

she originally started, before the advent of the "wonder
drugs." The only thing that can be done for these patients
is to give them good, devoted nursing care: but by now
the nurse has to some degree lost the knack of relying upon
her skill. Besides, even if she trusts herself she cannot trust
in the consistency of care among the rest of the personnel.

So the only thing she can do is to try to make the situation as safe as possible for everyone concerned. She gets
permission to transfer the patient to a single room, as far
from circulation as possible. She will give him paper dishes,
which can be discarded. She will perhaps discourage other
staff members from too much contact with the patient and
do the same herself, to reduce the possibility of cross-in-
fection.

We can understand the nurse's point of view, but what
does it do to the patient? He feels rejected, "unclean," a
menace to society, as patients with leprosy felt not very
long ago. Needless to say, such ideas about himself are not
conducive to a speedy and uneventful recovery.

What can the nurse do? I think she needs to request a
get-together with other nurses and her nurse administrator
or in-service person and openly raise the questions which
need clarification: Is the technique carried out at the moment safe? How can we go about finding this out? If it is,
how can we ensure that everybody who comes in contact
with patients follows the technique consistently? If it is
not, what other ways of dealing with infections should be
instituted? Physicians and bacteriologists may well be called
in for consultation. Tests can be set up to make sure that
the proposed solutions are effective.

Steps of that nature are being taken in many institutions,
but I know that in many others they are not, and the nurses
are merely disgruntled and afraid. It is not their intention,
but the patients have to pay for this by being rejected,
ignored, and neglected. My point is that care of contagious
patients is a nursing responsibility, hence the nurse must

insist on having, along with the responsibility, the rational authority (i.e., one based on scientific evidence) to make the care of these patients as safe as possible for everyone concerned. This in turn will free her emotionally to extend to the patient the interpersonal support which he badly needs. If the situation is such that the nurse cannot have responsibility in the decision making in such matters, in spite of her request for it, and instead is asked to follow prescribed routines for which she gets no explanations as to their rationale and safety, she is not only free, but in my opinion actually obliged, to leave the situation; or if this is impossible, to refuse to participate in a nursing practice which she as a licensed practitioner considers unsafe.

In this chapter we discussed the changes that have taken place in the care of patients with contagious illness and some of the reasons why these changes leave the nurse very uncomfortable about the possibility of spreading the disease. We have made some suggestions how the nurse can handle her discomfort to improve the situation, so that in spite of changed methods she can give safe and needed care to her patients.

Chapter 17
The Patient Who
Has Visitors
(Or: It's Not the Patient, It's His Family)

How many times have nurses made statements like this, "the patient is no trouble at all, it is his family who drive me out of my mind"? What is it that family members tend to do that makes life so hard for nurses? Well, for one thing, families exist. They are forever in the way when the nurse wants to do something for the patient. Families of ward patients are "better"; they will leave the bedside when they see the nurse approaching. But families of private patients seem to think "they own the place." The nurse often feels as if she were an intruder and practically has to apologize for giving care to the patient.

But this is not all. Families also tend to become emotional with sick patients. "They upset him" by their crying. Some will harass the nurse with questions like "How did he spend the night?" or "What did he eat for lunch today?"—questions which to her may appear irrelevant, considering the more serious issue of the patient's illness. As we have discussed in Chapter 4 and also Chapter 7, nurses do not like to be asked questions which as nurses they are not entitled to answer. Hence, a family member who calls up the private duty nurse of her critically ill relative and says, "You say he spent a quiet night—does that mean he is a little bit better today?" does not endear herself to the nurse. Nor, of course, does the nurse endear herself to the family member by just telling her that she is not saying anything one way or another (the patient is still on the critical list).

119

Then, there are family members who ask for silly little things such as ice cubes, even though they can see how busy the nurse is. In fact, she may be so busy that while asking them to get the ice cubes themselves from the utility room or the ward kitchen, she has forgotten that entrance to these rooms is forbidden to anyone who is not on the hospital staff.

Finally, there are the family members who attack the nurse verbally, but who imply they would love to do more than that, concerning their dissatisfaction with the care the patient is getting (meanwhile the nurse knows she has given her utmost to make this patient as comfortable as possible). These are examples of how family members are seen by many nurses.

And how are nurses seen by family members? They frequently see a grim or doll-like starched figure who enters and leaves the room wordlessly, at best with a noncommittal smile, in order to perform some more or less mysterious procedure. Her nod to the relatives leaves no doubt that they are to leave the room. What is she doing to the patient? What will it do for him? What is his condition—is he getting better, or worse? They do not dare ask, because they know that the most likely answer is that they should ask the doctor if they want information.

So they go out into the corridor, feeling helpless, wondering whether they did right in abandoning their charge to this formidable machinery, the hospital. Those who assumed quite a bit of responsibility before for their relatives who are now ill, as a wife would for her husband or a mother for her child, are liable to feel especially helpless now that the nurse has taken over so exclusively and efficiently. So they stand huddled in the corridor. There are rarely any chairs or benches in corridors, only in a far-off "visitors' room" to which they do not wish to go because they cannot expect the nurse to come there and notify them that she is finished with her procedure. They fight down their tears, which are a mixture of concern about the outcome of the illness, their own helplessness and their rage against the efficient machine in white who has taken over as if the patient had always belonged to her—as if they, the relatives, had never played any role in the patient's life. No wonder, then, if the patient's wife or mother finds a torn sheet or a spot of food on the patient's gown she will turn like a fury at the nurse and challenge the kind of care the patient is getting, for she herself could certainly do better than that.

What is the matter here? Why is it that in many hospitals mothers may not accompany their children to the ward but have to say good-bye at the elevator? And why is it that relatives of patients who are being treated in emergency rooms are asked to wait outside—and often to wait for hours before any word is given them as to the patient's condition, the treatment he is getting, and the chances for his immediate and long-range future? And when nurses do take time out to reassure the family, why are they often reprimanded for not using their time properly? Is it that the hospital sees itself as taking care of patients only? Is the family considered as something septic that must be removed from the patient just as his clothes and all of his belongings? It is right that the patient be the focus of attention, for after all he would not have come to the hospital if he had not been in dire need of its services. But does the fact of his hospitalization undo the fact that he is also a member of his family and has been one, for better or for worse, for longer than he has been a part of the hospital community?

I am sure that it is not the nurse's intention to create additional stress in one person (the relative), while she is doing her utmost in alleviating the suffering of another. And yet, by not giving the relatives an idea of what is going on, she does precisely that. I do not mean that she is to tell them what is wrong with the patient, what his treatment is, and what the prognosis of his illness is (see Chapter 7); this is the doctor's prerogative. But between just letting the relative fend for himself and giving him medical information, there are many things a nurse can say to reduce the relative's anxiety.

She can tell the relatives the doctor is seeing the patient, that it may take so-and-so much time until he will be able to talk with them (if it should take longer, she will let them know). She can say that she cannot give them any information as to the severity of the condition, but that the doctor will be in a position to do so after he has examined the patient and initiated treatment. Remarks of that nature may make all the difference between a relative who is self-possessed and cooperates with the hospital staff in doing what is best for the patient, and a relative who, because of having had to wait without clues as to what is going on, has developed a high degree of anxiety. In order to get some relief, he may well be exhibiting quite irrational behavior which obstructs the progress of care to the patient.

For example: A ten-year-old boy fell and has a profusely bleeding scalp wound. The mother, seeing all the blood and the child's pallor, is panicky when she brings him into the emergency room. The nurse and the doctor ask her to wait outside while they examine the child. The boy cries a little when the nurse starts cleaning out the injured area. The mother, in the corridor, walks up and down, ringing her hands, and also crying. Her anxiety mounts as she hears movement and voices in the room and does not know their meaning. Suddenly she hears her child call her, and without stopping to think, she opens the door to the emergency room. The child had not really called her—he is answering the doctor's questions. The mother feels embarrassed, for both the doctor and the nurse gesture to her to leave them to their work. What happened? The anxiety of the mother had reached such a high degree that she had to make use of irrational means to alleviate it (see also Chapter 14). A distortion of her perception has occurred: she has misinterpreted what the child was saying to suit her need for closeness with him. This phenomenon is called *illusion*.

Now, suppose the mother must wait longer. The nurse is shaving the injured area and preparing it to be sutured by the doctor. But the mother does not know this. She does not know either that the wound was really not big and that two or three stitches will do. Nor does she know that her child is getting local anesthesia, hence will not feel any pain. As she continues to wait, she hears the child cry out for her again. This time the child was not even talking; the perception was entirely imaginary on her part. Though not psychotic, this mother has had to resort to *hallucination* in order to come to grips with her feeling of mounting panic. Since she has been shown the door once, she does not dare to go back in again—and there is still no word from the doctor. Her anxiety continues to mount. As a result she suddenly gets the idea that the child has not only a bleeding head wound, but also may have a fractured skull. Since she does not hear anything, she *knows* that he has a fractured skull, that his life is in danger, that perhaps he is dying this very minute. And "this young doctor and his nurse won't let me be with him in his last moments—me, his mother!" So she storms into the room, ready to take the boy into her arms and to hold him there until it is all over.

By now the doctor and the nurse are really annoyed with her, and the doctor says rather sharply: "How many times do I have to ask you to wait until I call you?" She looks; the boy is all right, the blood is gone, he does not seem to have much pain. And to add insult to injury, he says; "Oh, mom, don't you hear what the doctor said?" (because he feels responsible for and embarrassed by his mother's behavior). And none of the participants know that the mother had, even if only for a brief period, a serious break with reality, that she became the victim of a *delusion* simply because she could not tolerate the uncertainty any longer.

As I mentioned before, I am sure that the nurse did not intend to contribute to the relative's panic; all she meant to do was to focus on the patient as her primary concern.

From what I have observed, it is quite common for nurses not only to focus on the patient rather than his family, but that they also tend to side with his needs versus those of the family. And so, by mothering the patient, as it were, they seem to become "mothers-in-law" to his relatives. They seem to feel the need of protecting the patient from his family. Granted, this is necessary sometimes, for visiting hours may prove to be quite exhausting to a patient, yet, in many cases it is the presence of the family that gives the patient the strength to continue to fight his battle toward health, that gives meaning to his life, and that gives him some inner peace in these strange, pain-harboring surroundings. Perhaps I am exaggerating: much progress has been made with visiting hours. They have been lengthened in many hospitals, especially in childrens' units. Yet many a nurse still conceives of them as a nuisance.

And yet, instead of being annoyed, all nurses could, as many do already, make more use of the family to give patient care. Not only would they themselves be less harassed by the amount of their work but the family would feel so much less helpless, knowing that they are contributing to the welfare of their loved one. They would also feel so much less guilty about being well themselves and standing by idly while their loved one may be struggling with death. I have a friend who invariably asks family members who complain about the care the patient is getting to help her in bathing him and changing his bedding. She makes sure that they have to do part of the hard physical labor involved in patient care. And invariably the family members feel useful, if tired, and have gained an appreciation of the care their loved one is receiving.

Perhaps one reason why it is hard for nurses to identify with family members of their patients is that they themselves are apt to have special privileges when a relative of theirs is hospitalized. They are usually allowed to enter the hospital and even the sickroom whenever they come, and they often are permitted to participate in the care the patient is getting. Hence they may find it hard to imagine what it is like if one does *not* have these privileges.

What is the nurse to do, though, if the family really irritates the patient? I think she will have to use her judgment in this as in all other situations. Will it really seriously harm the patient if the excitement continues? Or is this the kind of scene which sounds violent but is probably the way the patient and his spouse have been talking to each other ever since the honeymoon was over? In any case she might talk to the patient after visiting hours and assess what his reaction was to his wife's visit. If she does have to curtail visiting time because it is so indicated, she can make herself available both to the patient and his family, so that each can at least talk to *her* about their concerns. It is amazing how much a nurse can do, if she just listens and focuses her attention on what the patient's illness has done to the relative. A sure indication that it has done more than the relative is able to take is when the relative starts complaining about her symptoms (see Chapter 3), getting relief from anxiety by tying it to the body.

Precarious as it often may seem to the outsider, family life does seem to have an inherent balance. And when one member of the family is suddenly pulled out, this delicate balance may well be seriously upset and leave the others with reduced emotional resources—quite aside of the financial stress. Since all imbalance seeks to find a new equilibrium, it often happens that the family members outside the hospital find a new balance, one in which the patient himself is not included (see also Chapter 9). When he does return home after a prolonged illness, another imbalance occurs, and another adjustment for him *and* his family may be difficult and sometimes outright impossible, with the result that they and he tend to find a pretext that will let him return to the hospital. (We see this frequently with mental patients and with seriously disabled patients.)

In making herself available to the family as well as the patient, the nurse will facilitate the making of plans concerning referrals to helping agencies, if this should prove necessary. But even without a specific purpose, the nurse is giving the family members strength through her being there and her willingness to take them as people who are troubled. This in turn will give the nurse the opportunity to see the patient as a member of his home circle, to whom the stay in the hospital is only one, if serious, event of his life. Thus she will be able to see herself and her role toward the patient in the proper proportion, which in turn will increase her tolerance for the patient's family.

In this chapter we have discussed some ways in which the nurse sees the patient's family and some ways in which the family members see the nurse. We have taken a look at some of the problems nurses may have with relatives and vice versa. We looked at some of the unnecessary, and perhaps serious, anxiety which family members may have to suffer simply because there is not sufficient communication to them from the hospital staff. We have, finally, made some suggestions how the nurse can help in alleviating the family's plight, which in turn alleviates her plight with them.

Suggested Reading

Patients Have Families by Henry B. Richardson (Harvard University Press, 1945).

PART III:
SOME SOLUTIONS TO HAVING
PROBLEM PATIENTS

Chapter 18
What the Nurse Can Do
About Helplessness

In Part I we discussed some of the general reasons why nurses are apt to have problem patients. We found (Chapter 1) that by asking too much of herself and by setting up goals which cannot be reached because they are too high or because of an unsurmountable barrier that intervenes, a nurse may find herself in the throes of frustration. We found further (Chapter 2) that by aiming to please too many masters at the same time (the patient, the supervisor, the doctor, and the other staff nurses), a nurse may find herself practically immobilized by conflict. We found (Chapter 3) that, if she expects her patient to behave the way she thinks he should and the patient behaves differently, the nurse may be overwhelmed by anxiety. We found finally (Chapter 4), that as a result of being inadequately prepared to handle sophisticated questions from well-informed patients, and yet wanting to be able to answer, a nurse may feel utterly helpless.

As we looked at the various types of problem patients, we met up again and again with these four cardinal themes: frustration, conflict, anxiety, and helplessness. Remember these examples: The uncooperative patient who breaks hospital rules and leaves the nurse fuming with frustration; the flirtatious patient who insists that he wants the nurse's home phone number, with the result that the nurse is in conflict; the patient who does not want to get out of bed, even though he seems perfectly capable of doing so—a behavior not expected by the nurse, which evokes anxiety in her; the dying patient who asks her whether "this is the end," a question which may leave the nurse with a profound feeling of inadequacy and helplessness. There were other examples of the same nature: the adolescent who does not want to go to sleep; the old lady who soils herself the moment you have made her comfortable; the executive who treats the nurse as a servant; the professional who seems to look right through her; and many more.

In each instance we demonstrated that, unless the nurse saw a way to resolve the situation constructively, she would sooner or later be overcome by a profound feeling of helplessness, no matter whether the original situation had first resulted in frustration, conflict, or anxiety. As we stated in Chapter 4 and in many chapters in Part II, it is almost intolerable for adults to feel helpless. Hence they will convert this feeling into an attitude of hopelessness or an act of withdrawal; either of these will afford relief to the person feeling helpless, but neither will contribute much to the solution of the problem.

It is necessary for us, therefore, to take a good look at helplessness and to see whether we can avoid getting into this "bind" in the first place. As we saw in Chapter 4, a person feels helpless if he suddenly finds himself in a situation in which the competencies he had (or thought he had, we shall add here) no longer work. The recognition of this fact, or the surprise connected with it, seems to trigger an idea in the person that he is incapacitated not only in this one area but that this incapacitation has spread to his entire being. This idea results in perception of himself as totally inadequate, and this in turn seems to literally paralyze the individual's ability to act. In order to escape from this state of paralysis, the person will resort to the various mechanisms we have described in Chapter 4.

The question we have not raised so far is why the in-

ability to function in one little area (for instance, the failure
to know exactly what answer to give to a patient's questions)
should have such a devastating effect on a person. If we can
find an answer to this, we can perhaps also find a way to
prevent helplessness from occurring in the first place.

Karen Horney has said that people have three ways of being: the way they *think* they are (which is often the way others
have told them they are or the way they would like others to
see them), the way they *really* are, and, finally, the way they
could be if they realized their full potential. Now I shall try
to demonstrate that the closer these three ways of being are
to each other, the less need there will be for helplessness and
vice versa.

For example: I have a Spanish-speaking patient who
knows no English; I do not know any Spanish. The patient
is crying and I would very much like to understand what
this is all about, so that perhaps I can be of some service
to her. I look for an interpreter among the staff and the
patients but cannot find one. I report the matter to the
supervisor, who comes back after a while and states that
she has searched, but it so happens that at this moment there
is no one who speaks Spanish who can come down and talk
to my patient.

If the way I am, the way I think I am, and the way I
could be are pretty close together, I shall probably reason
the following way: This is too bad, but there is nothing I
can do about it at the moment. I am a pretty good nurse,
however, and I shall try to comfort this woman as best I
can with my presence, with my care, with my touch, with
gestures and smiles and by pointing to objects, until someone of her family comes who could serve as an interpreter. I
shall look at her dressing while I am with her, and I shall
palpate the area around it to check whether she has pain.
In order not to keep running into situations similar to this
one (which is likely to happen in view of the many Spanish-
speaking patients we are now getting), I will realize that it

will be more than worth while for me to take a course in Spanish as soon as I see my way clear to do so (i.e., as soon as I am through with the courses I am taking presently).

Although in this instance there has been a lack of competency in the area of verbal communication, there is no feeling of helplessness. I know what I can do and cannot do; and I also know what I would like to do and whether this is within the range of my present abilities or future potential. Now let us look at this situation when there is quite a discrepancy between what I think I am or can do, what I really am and can do, and what my potential is.

When the supervisor tells me that there is no one around at the moment who can talk with the patient, I become very upset. "But this patient needs someone to talk to *right now*," I tell her ("and I am not a good nurse in her or my eyes unless I can provide such a person," I think to myself). "Well, there isn't anybody at the moment," says the supervisor, and leaves me to my feelings which are anything but kind or peaceful.

What has happened here? Well, I have just had a terrible jolt to my picture of myself (or self-image as it is called). I had thought that I would be able to help this Spanish woman to communicate with me no matter what, but I had overestimated my capacities. Worse, I believed in this overestimate as the real me. Now my bluff has been called. Since what I thought was real has dissolved into nothing, how can I trust my other capacities, which I thought were real too? Perhaps they too are just figments of my imagination.

Although I probably do not reason this way consciously, this is the kind of reasoning which has gotten me into the state of helplessness I am in now. I do not trust myself, since I am now different from the way I thought I was. Since I am so badly shaken in what I expected of myself, I respond with a great deal of anxiety (see Chapter 3). In order to get rid of the anxiety and to mobilize myself out of the paralysis of helplessness, I become very angry at my supervisor. If she had tried harder, she could have rounded up someone to help out. There just *must* be someone some place, I think; it is imperative that someone talk to this poor distressed woman in her own language.

So I leave the floor (and all the patients on it) and run upstairs, sure that I shall find an interpreter. But as I am about halfway up, the supervisor intercepts me. "What are you doing up here?" she asks. I tell her what my errand is. Now she begins to get angry, too, and lets me know that it is high time for me to see an ear doctor, for obviously I have not heard what she told me just a few minutes ago.

I turn back, smoldering and discouraged. I sit at my desk for the rest of the day and let my aides answer the bells. I never once go back to my patient. I am mad at her too: why couldn't she have learned English before she came to the hospital? How does she expect me to help her if we cannot understand each other? I feel tired, helpless, and hopeless: "Oh, what's the use—you just can't win. . . ."

What happened here? I saw myself in the role of "savior" without stopping to realize that at this time the necessary skills for "saving" were not available. By wanting to be what I was not able to be at the time, I neglected to look at what I *was* able to be, i.e., a good nurse who had instead of verbal skills other comforting measures at her disposal. Thus I got in trouble with my supervisor, neglected the patient, and, in a way prevented myself from recognizing my potential for at least future growth and competency. I did not see, or ignored, the possibility that I might learn some Spanish and some day might not have to get into such situations, at least not with Spanish-speaking patients.

Do you see my point? Helplessness can be avoided, if one is pretty clear about, and can accept the limitations of, what one can do and what one cannot do and what one will be able to do, with additional preparation.

Here is another example to amplify my point. Suppose

I am a staff nurse on day duty. The patient I am assigned to, a sixty-year-old woman with hemiplegia resulting from a cerebrovascular accident, asks me whether I saw a certain TV program the night before. I tell her that I have not seen it and ask her why she wants to know this. Instead of answering me, she begins to have tears in her eyes and points to the box of tissues at her nightstand.

Gradually I can draw her out about what is going on. The essence of her story is that this particular program is her favorite and she had to miss it, because the nurse on evening duty has the habit of putting all patients to bed at four P.M. and will not help them get up after that, because she has "enough work to do as is." Since the patient had no TV set in her room, she just had to miss the show.

As I receive this information, I have the choice of feeling completely helpless with impotent rage or of using my competencies for the patient's benefit. I can feel most indignant about this incident and tell the evening nurse what I think of her; this will not alter the situation, because I really have no jurisdiction over her tour of duty. All that this maneuver can accomplish is to antagonize this nurse more than she already is (for reasons of her own), with the probable result that she will ask me to mind my own business. This in turn will make me feel even more helpless than I already do feel by just having listened to the patient. I could also report this nurse to the director of nursing, but the chances are that I shall again be asked to mind my business, because nurses for evening duty are scarce nowadays. I can also try to convince the patient that the evening staff has so much work to do that she must have a little understanding. This may be true, but should patients really be convinced that their routine depends on the way the staff can manage their work? I can also shrug my shoulders, or change the subject.

Any one of these procedures will leave me more helpless and will not help the patient either. I can also, the moment the patient speaks to me, realize that this is an issue which is beyond my jurisdiction, i.e., beyond my competency to be of help, insofar as the patient and the evening nurse are concerned. But instead of being flooded with helplessness (and I shall only feel helpless if I have assumed that I can save all patients all heartaches and then find out that I cannot), I can immediately ascertain in what areas I am *not* helpless. I find that I can certainly *listen* to the patient and let her express her own feelings of disappointment and grievance. In fact, I can help *her* to understand about helplessness (just as I learned to understand it, in Chapter 4).

I can help her to understand why she feels the way she does at the moment; i.e., I can help her to identify her present feeling of helplessness and let her see how it resulted from frustration. I can help her to find the component parts of her feelings and can help her to consider alternative ways of dealing with them in the future. If the nurse on evening duty proves to be an unsurmountable barrier to her goal of watching TV, what else can be done about goal and barrier? Many alternatives exist and the patient will select the one most suitable to her.

I can also help her to come to grips with the areas in which she must acknowledge limits of her powers and the areas in which no one can take away her autonomy—for instance, her personal rights, her thoughts, and a basic understanding of what is going on in an institution.

As I put this competency to use, I suddenly do not feel helpless at all. For I am making use of what I can do to the degree to which I can put it to use (instead of focusing on what I cannot do), and both the patient and I have grown from this experience.

I hope that these two examples have made clear my point that it is possible not to be overwhelmed by helplessness. There are, however, occasions on which we have, without knowing it, overestimated our capacities or where circumstances suddenly arise for which we have not been prepared. In such cases we shall, of course, have to acknowledge that we have been taken unawares and are, as a result, helpless at the moment. Yet instead of getting frantic about it, and thus spreading the inner paralysis, we can try to ascertain how far the damage already has progressed, and which capacities we still can use.

Since we have covered the solution to helplessness if it actually occurs, in Chapter 4, I would like to go on now to some of the other possible solutions to problems posed in Part I, namely how to get out of frustration, conflict, and anxiety. These we shall discuss in the following three chapters. In the final chapter we shall again turn to helplessness, to see whether there is not *some* way in which we can get help to strengthen our own capacities.

Chapter 19

What The Nurse Can Do About
Her Expectations of Herself

In Chapter 1 we suggested that many a nurse is liable to become frustrated because she expects more of herself than she can deliver. Some of the reasons for such high expectations and resulting frustrations are: The nurse, because she is so highly motivated, may tend to neglect acknowledging her limitations as a human being and, therefore, may make inhuman demands on herself. She may tend to limit the concept of "helping" to the meanings of "curing" or at least "getting results," and thus may find that what she can do for some patients seems to be very limited. Further, frustration results when a person sets up a goal which cannot be attained because of an intervening barrier which blocks the approach to the goal. As a result the energy which was originally directed toward the goal bounces against the barrier and is converted into anger which becomes focused on the barrier. Or it may be displaced toward another person or object or goes back in reverse direction against oneself. The end result is likely to be helplessness, resignation, and eventual indifference.

Let us look now at the various alternatives open if one wants to reach a goal but finds a barrier blocking it. It may well be that the barrier lies in the simple fact that the goal is so high that the person will never be able to reach it through his own efforts alone, unless he develops wings (which even in the space age is unlikely to happen). In this case the most reasonable choice would be to lower the goal to an attainable height. Perhaps the barrier is such that it will not or cannot yield to any direct attack, no matter how forceful. In this case one may have to surmount the barrier by climbing over it, through physical or intellectual efforts, or circumvent it by going around it rather than attacking it. Perhaps neither of these alternatives is possible. Then the barrier will have to be accepted for what it is, and that implies that the goal beyond it may have to be abandoned or moved somewhere else where there is no barrier between the person and the goal.

The strength of the force which wishes to reach the goal also needs to be considered. If there is a great deal of energy in the goal-directed force, it may be able to knock down the most resistant barrier, if it tries hard enough. If it is weak, it had better watch out, lest it exhausts itself in attempting to climb over, circumvent, or attack the barrier. Perhaps the goal-directed force is not very powerful but is as enduring as a little stream of water, which given time, can undermine the most solid rock.

How aware is the nurse of all these factors? Does she weigh each against the other and come to some rational conclusion? Or does she merely find out that she is frustrated, after she has been forced to seek aid for the bumps she accumulated on her forehead after repeated blind assaults against the barrier?

Each nurse will have to substitute the concrete situational items for the more general terms "goal" and "barrier" and "force," but the problem to be solved will be the same, just as substituting numbers for letters in algebra does not alter the basic problem.

Let us go back to one of the main reasons for the nurse's functioning, i.e., her wanting to be a nurse of top quality with no human shortcomings. There is nothing wrong with this goal—somehow we would all like to reach it. But at the same time we must know that though we shall never be able to reach it completely, just because we are human, there is nothing to stop us from getting closer and closer to it. Thus, I think that one is never the good nurse one would like to be, but one is rather always in the process of becoming a better nurse than one was a year ago or a month ago or even one day ago. The more one can accept inevitable fluctuations in the quality of one's work, instead of being unhappy about them, the more energy one will have available for eventual improvement.

For example, many women cannot help being irritable during the last week before their period; they are also often slower-moving during this time. Or if a nurse is worried about her husband's fidelity or a sick child at home, she may well be less efficient than usual. I know that patients will grant her these human failings, as long as she acknowledges them, i.e., admits that today she is a little slow, or a little irritable, or not quite as efficient as usual. She need not tell the patient the reasons for her behavior, however, nor should she demand his indulgence. If the nurse feels that she is less efficient on a given day, she can ask to be given additional help or she can try to delegate some of her responsibilities to others.

Do I hear some of my readers object to this statement? "Ask for additional help? They never give you help. Nurses work their fingers to the bone and do not even get a 'thank you' for it." Now, who do you mean by "they"? Your head nurse, your supervisor, your director of nursing, your administrator? And who is "you"—me? Or do you mean yourself? If you do, please stick with it ("me" when you talk of yourself), otherwise you as an entity may get lost in the shuffle. How do you know that "they" never give help? Have you tried to find out—have you asked for help? Have you stated flatly that you cannot carry out your assignment alone, because it is beyond what you can do at this particular day or in general? Perhaps you have, I do not know. And you may have gotten into difficulty because of it. . . .

But this is why nurses as a group will have to come to grips before long with the taking of responsibility for the amount of work they can and should safely do (see also Chapters 12 and 22). Perhaps one of the reasons for not having done so yet lies (as outlined in Chapter 2) with the fact that so many nurses wish so much to be appreciated by their fellow men, that they will go along with any task given to them, whether it be a reasonable request or not.

Another important reason for not taking responsibility for determining the workload may lie in the fact that nurses are such devoted and highly motivated people that they are liable to feel very guilty if they do stand up for reasonable limits. For example, suppose a floor is not covered sufficiently and the nurse from the other floor is asked to take charge of two floors. I am sure that she will gladly consent if she can do it without neglecting her own patients, even if it means that she will have to use all her resources to do the job. But if she feels that by going along with this request, she may neglect her own patients, and will not be able to care adequately for either floor, and therefore shows some resistance to this request, her guilt feelings that she is unfair to the patients can be easily aroused. She will tend to go along with the request, in spite of her misgivings, because she does not wish to be selfish and unfair. And yet hospital staffing is not really her responsibility—or is it? Besides, if as a result of her taking care of two floors an act of negligence should occur, she as a licensed practitioner will be held liable for it. Also, if by taking on more than she can reasonably deliver, the nurse becomes curt and irritable toward staff or patients, she will most likely have to account for this behavior to her superiors later on. And the responsibility for having taken on the extra load will be entirely hers. Then it will be too late to be unhappy about the "unfair" treatment she is getting, for the blame will be on her.

This is why I think the nurse might as well determine herself the limits of what she can reasonably and safely accomplish. She cannot let her devotion be the substitute for better personnel policies and higher salaries; not for any moral reasons, but for purely practical and professional ones.

Will the nurse be fired for saying no, when saying yes would be irresponsible on her part? I do not know this. I doubt it, because using her has been merely a way of least resistance for her poor supervisor who is supposed to keep the institution running and has not enough staff to run it with. But if one nurse says no, and other nurses say no, when unsafe requests are made of them, the supervisor will have to take *her* stand, too, concerning the running of hospital wards with insufficient personnel. If the supervisors all do this, the director of nursing will have to take a stand about the number of patients who can be serviced by a certain number of personnel, and somehow or other things will change because they *have* to change.

Suppose the nurse does get fired because she refuses to do what, in her professional opinion, is unsafe practice. I think that in this case she has recourse to the support of her nursing organization. The practitioners within their nursing organization have already spelled out the functions, standards, and qualifications of the various levels and areas of practice, materials which are available to anyone for the asking. But a further step needs to be taken by the licensed practitioner, i.e., to set up standards for the time necessary for the care she gives. The question is how many patients needing such and such an amount of care can be served by one practitioner in a given amount of time?

One nurse alone cannot do this, for she has very little say-so in a complex institution such as our hospitals are nowadays. If she does make an attempt of this nature, the chances are that she will merely become unpopular or that she will be asked to resign since she obviously cannot cope with the workload. But, if several or all practitioners are convinced that it is up to them and not up to the administration to set down the minimum requirements for care given according to prescribed professional standards, they can, in cooperation with their head of nursing service, arrive at some tentative statements, which then will have to be verified in practice.

In considering the time the nurse needs for each patient, she may wish to specify how much of this time is actual nursing and how much time goes into functions which could also be carried out by non-nurses. If she is to take care of more patients than she can reasonably do justice to the way things are set up now, perhaps someone else can take over the non-nursing functions.

Some nurses do not like this idea, however. They do not feel comfortable for long periods right at the bedside, perhaps because they feel so inadequately prepared in interpersonal skills and yet know that the patient is entitled to their skill in this area. These nurses prefer to work for the patient indirectly, as it were. They would like to give him his treatments, check out his orders for him, make rounds with the doctor, and order supplies and medications.

It seems to me that reasonable arrangements could be made to delegate these functions to the nurses who like to take them on, and thus free nurses who like direct patient contact to give "pure" patient care to as many patients as they can give it to without lowering standards for each (1).

A nurse may say that this is all well and good but she never sees her director of nursing; it is almost impossible to get to her. This nurse can talk to other staff nurses about this, and she and they can jointly ask for meetings with the director of nursing to discuss the matter. She can talk about it in her nursing organization and with her colleagues work out some general plans there which can then be submitted to her director of nursing for consideration, with the understanding that modifications will have to be made for each individual setting.

Frustration occurs, then, when a nurse attempts to do the impossible upon request from others. It can occur just as easily when a nurse attempts to do the impossible in light of her innate capacities. If she is a slow and deliberate person and does not like to rush but accepts a position in an emergency room, she will soon be frustrated because most of her energies will go into mobilizing herself and she will always be many steps behind what she is supposed to accomplish. Or if a nurse who loves to give direct patient care but,

for economic and prestige reasons, decides that she will become a teacher, she will be most frustrated as she watches
her students' awkward attempts at mastering the art of
nursing.

The point I am trying to make is that each individual
has a unique contribution to make to his society. If he can
find out what this contribution is and if it is possible for
him to make his unique contribution, his energies will be
fully released in the work. If on the other hand he does
something which goes against his grain or his personality
make-up, most of his energy will be used up in overcoming
resistance against activity alien to his self. Also, doing what
is right for oneself is enjoyable, while doing what goes
against one's inner nature is distasteful to a person.

Now how does one know what one is cut out to do? The
possibilities are really not infinite in practice although they
may be so in theory. They have to do with a person's background, the choices he has been exposed to, and his abilities.
Out of this range the possibilities will be narrowed down
further by the opportunities available and the influences
prevailing upon the person's choice at a particular time. The
final choice will be in accord with what the person feels is
right for him. We shall have more to say on this topic in
the next chapter. For those who are interested, I suggest
the book by Victor Frankl, *The Doctor and the Soul,* in
which the idea of unique contributions is discussed quite
extensively (2).

We can summarize by saying that there are ways of
coping with frustration if one can assess the relationship
between goal, barrier, and force. One can avoid a great deal
of frustration if by and large one adheres to reasonable
standards for the amount of work one can produce (in spite
of attempts by others to appeal to one's sense of duty, which
triggers uncomfortable guilt feelings that have to be appeased
by taking on the additional burden) ; and if one tries to find
a place in which one can make the contribution which is,
given a variety of factors, most suitable to one's personality.

Chapter 20
What the Nurse Can Do About Wishing to Please Everybody

In Chapter 2 we discussed the fact that a nurse may be in conflict by aiming to please and at the same time aiming to do what she thinks is right. As we indicated, this may mean that she is sometimes trying to go in two opposite directions at once, with the result that she may find herself stuck in the middle and immobilized. We noted further that the nurse will be able to move again once she can make a choice between these two goals or decides upon a third goal. We differentiated between goals which lie in the area of security (such as the goal to be liked) and goals which lie in the direction of satisfaction (to do a professional job according to the standards which the nurse has set for herself).

We said that the nurse's decision to move in one direction or the other may depend on the strength of her needs at the moment, on the importance of the matter at hand, and on the support she is getting from the outside. We said, finally, that her main problem is not so much the decision *per se* but to recognize that she is in conflict and to know what her different goals are so that she can come to a decision. Therefore the alternatives of action are less important than an awareness of the hidden goals behind each alternative.

The question is *not* whether to force an oxygen tube on a resistive dyspneic patient or to report the patient's refusal to the doctor; whether to answer first the bell of an influential private patient who is not very sick or that of a ward patient who is very sick; or whether to disagree with one's colleagues about the interpretations of a patient's behavior or to go along with them so they won't think one knows it all. The question is rather: "What is *behind* the alternatives of action?" Thus, for our first example the question may be: "What am I really trying to get at by forcing the oxygen tube on this patient? And what am I aiming at if I do not do so, but instead call the doctor back?"

There are a multitude of possible answers. Here are just a few: "I would like to save this patient's life." Or "I am the one who knows what is best for the patient." "He does not know what he is doing, I must think for him." "The doctor told me to, so I had better do it—he knows best and will be angry if I do not follow his orders." I am sure you can think of many more.

If the nurse listens carefully to herself, she will be able to evaluate each of these answers: "I want to save his life, but will I if he struggles and uses up more oxygen in the struggle than I could possibly let him have through the tube?" Or "Who's need am I meeting in insisting that I know what is best for him, mine or this sick patient's?" or "What will happen to me if the doctor does get angry? Will I get fired? And, if I do? Have I really done wrong by not forcing this weak old man? I know that I can not reason with him, because he is so confused. Perhaps the doctor can give him some sedation, then the oxygen will be no problem. . . ."

Do you see that by examining the various goals, a decision has emerged, by itself almost. The nurse does what she *knows* is *right* for her to do. She can defend it, and although she may not like them, she is really not afraid of possibly unpleasant consequences.

The reader may rightly object that these are really very many questions to ask oneself in a hurry. I agree. But usually,

I think, one has only to leave oneself open to these questions: the asking and the answers will come up, almost simultaneously. For a person who has practiced such an approach, the answer may well come instantaneously.

Of course, to do this is a great deal easier for someone who from childhood on has been allowed to make decisions in matters which were within his province and his ability. Such a person will have developed a "self" which can make the choices which are right for himself and are usually rational in nature.

Other people have either had to make too many difficult decisions too early in life, or else have rarely had an opportunity to make any. They will find it harder to do so when they are grown up and may have a tendency to look upon others for the answers. Yet, if they follow others' suggestions, they will still not be sure whether they have made the right decision.

I do not mean that the person who decides by trusting his judgment always makes the right decision. He may err considerably and dangerously. But he has done what he felt was right; he has acted in the best faith, his act was the best he could do in the light of his best judgment. The other person listens to someone who may be right or not; he listens to someone else, who may give the opposite opinion. Now which one is he to choose? The choice is his, in the end.

Yet many people feel they cannot make a choice on their own; according to the literature, this is true of more and more people nowadays (1, 2). Such a person will say point blank that he would like to make the choice but he really does not know what he wants. Yes, he hears a tiny little voice which tells him somewhere from the pit of his stomach to do this or that, but can he trust this voice? There is another voice in his ear, a superior or commanding voice which says "Do as I tell you, otherwise you will be sorry." Also, there is some confusion between the little voice in the pit of the stomach and another little devilish voice, somewhere in the temples or in the back of the neck, which says: "Oh, gee, I'd love to do that instead."

Now which one of all these voices is he to trust, if they all talk at the same time and are equally strong? I cannot prove it, but as far as I know, it is the voice in the pit of the stomach (the region of the solar plexus) that belongs to the "self," which makes the best judgment for oneself. It is the voice which will from all available choices pick the right one. This will not necessarily be the one that will be most liked by others or even the one that will be liked most by the person himself; yet it will be the best answer for the situation. And each time a person can follow the advice of the little voice in the stomach region, this little voice will become stronger and therefore more audible and forceful.

Now let us enlarge upon this picture. These three voices are not isolated from each other, and the voice in the stomach is well informed about the wishes of the other two. There will be occasions when it will be in complete agreement with one or both other voices. For example, after a day of hard, satisfying work, it will suggest that the nurse sit down in an easy chair with her feet up, a good book to read, and perhaps a long cool drink. The voice in her ear will say, "You have been a good girl today, you deserve this rest." And the little devil in the temples will say, "Oh, this feels good, just what I wanted."

Now suppose the nurse has worked hard and is to get up early tomorrow. Yet in order to get "something out of life," she decides to go dancing in the evening, in spite of the voice in the pit of the stomach that tells her that she is really too tired, and in spite of the voice in her ears which tells her she will be sorry in the morning. So on top of feeling tired, she is also liable to feel guilty and thus unable to fully enjoy the dance, and the fatigue may last through the next day.

Suppose, on the other hand, she listens to the voice in

her ears that says she must rest up at any price, because
she has a heavy day ahead tomorrow. She goes along with
this voice, even though the voice in the solar plexus region
and the little devil in the brain say that they would like to
sit up for a while and read, just so that they can receive
back some of what they have given out during the day. She
finds that even though she goes to sleep, she does not feel
refreshed the next day: she feels empty and dissatisfied with
the drudgery of her life.

Do you get the point? I am not saying that a nurse should
not go dancing, nor am I saying that she should not go to
sleep early, if she feels tired. I am saying that it will be easier
for her to make decisions if she listens to all her inner
voices, but learns to trust the one which seems to come from
the center of her being. In time she will find that her choices,
if not always right, are consistent with her personality and
the task at hand. If she has erred, she has erred in good faith,
and although, perhaps, she will not always be popular, she
will be first respected, then liked by her patients and
coworkers.

Some nurses may find that, no matter how hard they
listen, they still cannot differentiate which voice comes from
where and which one they are to follow. I think these
nurses may find it helpful if they can find a reliable outside
source (not somebody who has an ax to grind, because this
person would support the wrong, the "ear" voice) who
will help them find their "stomach" voice and will support
them until they can recognize it themselves, trust it, and
follow it. I can assure you that once you are familiar with
this voice and have learned to respect it and follow it, you
will feel close to being a person who has found her place
and is making her unique contribution to this world and
thus has found fulfillment (see also Chapter 19). Work
then will stop being a series of pitfalls of little conflicts into
which the nurse falls one by one (as soon as she has climbed

out of one, the next one has engulfed her). It will be a challenge to exercise her talents and skills for her own and her patients' satisfaction.

Suggested Reading

Motivation and Personality by A. H. Maslow (Harper, 1954), chapters 12 and 13.
On Becoming a Person by Carl Rogers (Houghton, Mifflin, 1961).

Chapter 21
What the Nurse Can Do About
Her Expectations of Others

In Chapter 3 we discussed the fact that, by virtue of their preparation, nurses may tend to expect patients to conform to the values which have proven so important in our culture for the preservation or the regaining of health. Since the nurse tends to have such definite expectations as to how patients should act to get well or stay well and since she has learned to be so convinced of her own importance as the doctor's executive in showing the patient what is right for him, she is liable to become quite shocked if she encounters behavior which runs counter to her expectations or behavior which challenges her authority. This being shocked when one's expectations are not met or one's prestige needs are threatened is called anxiety.

We described anxiety as a most uncomfortable state to be in, a state of felt danger, from an unknown enemy coming from an unknown direction, out to threaten one's integrity and sense of security. We stated that, since anxiety is so uncomfortable, one tends to convert it into various other reactions (such as anger or detachment or righteousness or physical symptoms) before one is even fully aware of its presence. We stated that a perhaps more painful but certainly more constructive way of handling anxiety is to recognize it as an indication of the need to re-evaluate our expectations from ourselves and from others. In order to do this we shall need to ask ourselves what we did expect and what happened instead, and what this difference meant to us. This procedure will help us to understand some of the reasons why we became anxious. In addition, it will help if we can learn to expect a variety of behavior from our patients—just as we never quite know in what mood we shall find the other party when we make a phone call. We expect a certain *range* of behavior as we make the call, which lies within the boundaries of what we know about the other person. We can do similarly with what we expect of a patient's behavior.

The range will roughly be limited by the patient's illness, his cultural and socio-economic background, his position in life, his age, and his personality (which is a result of his family background and his own constitution).

Since the nurse can know very little about the patient when he comes in, she will be in a better position to make predictions the better she is informed about each of these categories in general. That is, how *do* patients with a certain illness behave? Do they all act the same way or are there variations? How do Italians in general react to hospitalization? What does illness mean to them? What are the variations in their behavior, or do all Italians act alike? And so on. (We have raised some of these questions in Chapters 9, 11, 12, 13, 14, and 15).

If a patient still acts very differently from the way a nurse can assume he will act in view of all the expected variables mentioned above, she will still become anxious. But in this case, she will be glad of this inner warning signal, because there is good reason for her alarm. This patient's behavior is not appropriate to himself nor the situation; it is out of context, as it were. This strange behavior may be an indication that his wholeness as a person has been put to too serious a test and that he is in the process of losing his hold on reality. It is not up to the nurse to determine that this is actually so; it is definitely up to her to report this matter immediately, before it becomes too late and the patient does something desperate in his search for just any kind of integrity (see also Chapter 8).

Here is an illustration. Many years ago I lived in a nurses' residence. One evening, the nurse who lived in the next room came in and asked for some aspirins because, as she said, she had a cold. She then sat down on my bed and began to talk. After a while she left and went back to her room. Although her physical condition did not warrant any great concern on my part, I found myself repeatedly going into her room to check up on how she was feeling. At each of my visits I sat down and listened some more to her talking. I did not know why I was doing it, I just felt I had to.

After a few hours of this, i.e., several visits later, it became apparent to me that there was something strange about the content of her talk. It made sense and yet it did not, and it was incongruous both with the person I had known before and with the physical condition she was suffering from. I had a suspicion that I was witnessing a "breakdown," something I had never seen before. And so I told her that I was going to make an appointment for her to be seen right away in the emergency room, because she was not well and needed help immediately. I told her that I would go with her and that I would stay with her until the doctor could see her.

My suspicion was right. If it had not been for my response of anxiety to her incongruous behavior, i.e., her behaving differently from the range of behavior I could have anticipated from knowing her and also from knowing about colds, something tragic might have happened. It turned out later that she had had strong suicidal impulses. But this way she was treated in time.

Do you see what I am trying to say? If your expectations are merely that another person conform to the way you want him to behave, you will be thrown by any deviation on his part and will have your hands full in trying to cope with your own anxiety.

If, on the other hand, you can gradually learn to have reasonable expectations which will be guided by what you know about the various criteria which are liable to influence your patient's behavior, you will be comfortable if he acts within this expected range of behavior. If you suddenly do become anxious, you may reasonably assume that your anxiety has been triggered by inappropriate behavior, and that it should be taken as a warning sign that something unusual is going on, an indication for immediate expert evaluation of the situation.

There are, of course, certain events which can happen which are so unexpected and so out of context to the nurse's usual way of life that she may find herself unable to utilize her anxiety as a cue for appropriate action, but instead finds herself overcome with panic. This may well happen if an unexpected serious (or pleasant) event occurs to someone close to her, or herself.

Since panic makes rational thinking practically impossible, the nurse will need to reduce her anxiety by mechanical means until she reaches the level which will permit her to examine the situation more closely. Physical activity is useful here and, if possible, getting away from the place where the anxiety started. Thus, a brisk walk can be very helpful. But sometimes the nurse cannot get away, in fact she must stay where she is and perform perhaps life-saving functions. In this case it will help to concentrate on the concrete task and to spell it out for herself step by step. This will reduce the anxiety to manageable proportions and will prevent the nurse from doing something which she might regret later on. The popular saying that one should count to ten when upset before going into some irrational action is based on the same principle.

I have no doubt that, with adequate preparation, nurses can be as expert in handling emotional stress in others as they now are in physical emergencies. I would like to examine the reasons why most nurses are such experts in handling physical emergencies and then see whether we cannot draw some conclusions for the handling of inter-personal situations.

I have seen again and again that no matter what emer-gency arises, whether it be hemorrhage, or cardiac arrest, or a bad fall, nurses are right on the job and do what is right without hesitation and without faltering. For what others may see as emergencies has become a part of the nurse's anticipated range of functioning. What are the ingredients of this proficiency on the nurse's part?

First of all, nurses have learned about symptoms: they are informed about their nature, under what general condi-tions they may occur, and what the reasons and precipitating factors for their occurrence are. Nurses have further learned how to recognize these symptoms and what effects they will produce on the organism.

Second, nurses have learned about emergency measures. They know which one to apply to what symptom and the principles or reasons for doing so, and this will help them to improvise, should it be necessary.

Third, in addition to their theoretical knowledge and readiness to anticipate the symptom, nurses have had the necessary amount of practice and actual drill in spotting the symptom the moment it occurs and in applying the neces-sary emergency measure without having to stop and think about the procedure. This is most useful when there is a great deal of excitement or confusion around the situation, for the anxiety aroused by such situations would make thinking practically impossible (see Chapter 10) .

But besides having these three areas of competency (knowing about the symptom, knowing about emergency measures, and having skills in both areas) a nurse can func-tion so safely and efficiently in physical emergencies because she feels *secure* in her knowledge and skill, because she has, in midst of chaos and excitement, a concrete task to focus on, and because this task and she as the person who executes it are vitally needed to the other human being (see also Chapter 16).

Is there any reason why a similar proficiency on the part of the nurse could not be developed in the area of interpersonal relationships? And could not the same ingredients for proficiency apply as those applying to physical emergencies? Let us consider this, and compare an instance of hematemesis with an attack of anxiety.

Let us look at the symptom first. The nature of the symptom in hematemesis is a vomiting of blood. The nature of anxiety is a feeling of fear of an unknown enemy. The general conditions under which hematemesis may occur are peptic ulcers, esophageal varices, etc. The general conditions when anxiety occurs are when a person has certain expectations and certain prestige needs, and when a person puts complete trust in certain or all of his competencies, whether they be real or imagined (see Chapter 18).

The reason for the symptom in case of hematemesis may be the erosion of a blood vessel wall by an ulcer or a sudden pressure within the blood vessel which may break an already weakened wall. The reason for anxiety may be the fact that one's expectations or prestige needs are not met by others or that there has been a sudden switch in efficacity of one's competencies.

The precipitating factor in hematemesis may have been a heavy, spiced meal, or a blow on the nose, or an argument with one's landlord. The precipitating factor in a patient's anxiety may have been his inability to get answers to his questions, with a resulting unbearable state of uncertainty (see Chapters 4, 7, and 17); or the humiliation of his dignity and social status through hospital routine or through the invasion of his privacy by certain hospital procedures. Another precipitating factor may be his sudden awareness of the loss of competencies he had heretofore called his own, such as the loss of an organ or a function such as walking (see Chapter 10).

Let us continue with our comparison. How does the nurse recognize hematemesis? There may or may not be a period of nausea and after that the patient will vomit bright red or coffee-ground fluid. The nurse will probably be able to tentatively differentiate hematemesis from hemoptysis (for example), because the vomitus will probably contain food particles or bile and there will be retching and a flushed face rather than coughing and cyanosis (although sometimes it may not be possible to differentiate between the two).

How will the nurse recognize anxiety? She will notice a slight or considerable restlessness, an increase or decrease in the flow of speech, a scattering of the topics discussed or a narrowing down of them to seemingly unimportant details. She will notice changes in the patient's skin color, such as flushing or blotching of the skin or an increasing pallor. She will also notice beads of perspiration above the upper lip or over the entire face, clammy palms, and staining of the clothing under the armpits from perspiration. She may also find that the patient has to wet his lips continuously with his tongue or that he drinks repeatedly sips of water.

How can the nurse differentiate anxiety from pain or shock? This may be difficult sometimes, because pain is often associated with anxiety and anxiety is often associated with shock. But if her observational skills have been trained, the nurse will recognize any physical attitude which may point to pain rather than anxiety. She can also ask the patient, since he is conscious, whether he feels pain and where.

What are the effects of hematemesis and anxiety on the organism? If the hemorrhage cannot be stopped the patient will probably become weak, restless, dyspneic; his pulse rate will increase, the pulse beat will become weaker, his skin will become pale and clammy—in short, he will go into shock. If the hemorrhage continues and no help is forthcoming, the patient is liable to die from the effect of anoxia to his vital organs.

Since anxiety is so difficult for a person to tolerate (see Chapter 3), the patient's system will soon defend itself against it (in fact, it is hard to differentiate between symptom and defense against the symptom in the emotional and the physiological area. For example, an increased pulse rate is a symptom of hemorrhage, and is also a reparative mechanism, making up for lack of volume by frequency of circulation). Some of the defense mechanisms (or effects of anxiety on the person) will be restlessness, overtalkativeness, withdrawal, anger, aloofness, and, in severe cases, bewilderment, denial (see Chapter 10), and even perceptual and thought distortions (as described in Chapter 17).

As noted, the second major reason for a nurse's proficiency in coping with physical emergencies is the fact that she knows which emergency measure to apply to what symptom, and what the reasons behind such measure are. In the case of hematemesis, after seeing that the doctor is notified, she will put the patient to rest, stay with him, and try to calm him. She will perhaps ask that an icebag be brought and put on his stomach region. She will withhold everything by mouth until the doctor has seen the patient, but she will wipe the patient's lips with a moist cloth or a piece of ice. She will put extra blankets on the patient and, if the bleeding had been copious, or if he seems to be going into shock, she may lower the head-end of the bed and raise the foot-end. She will take the patient's pulse and blood pressure at frequent intervals. She may ask that someone prepare all the emergency medications should the doctor ask for them, and that someone fill out all the necessary slips for blood typing, in case a transfusion should be required. Since she knows what is behind the symptom, she can anticipate actions appropriate to consequences of the symptom.

Similarly, the nurse can anticipate the consequence of anxiety. She can assess its level and the appropriate measures, as we described in Chapter 10. If the patient is in a panic, she will stay with him and give him some concrete directions.

Later she needs to listen, mainly, so that the patient can discharge some anxiety by talking, and only after the anxiety has subsided considerably can she help the patient to figure out what it was all about in the first place. As discussed in Chapter 9, the nurse can let the patient describe the situation until the concept and its component parts emerge clearly. Then she can point out the component parts to him and can show him how, by juggling all or some of them, he can avoid becoming anxious in the future or can reduce his anxiety. (She had better do this before the anxiety has subsided entirely, because by then the patient may feel too comfortable to want to know. And that is a pity, in a way. It seems to me that if one has to go through a most uncomfortable experience, one might as well find out why it happened so that one may gain some assurance that it will not have to happen again—at least if one had anything to do with its occurrence in the first place.)

Just as the nurse keeps an eye on patients with peptic ulcers or cancer of the stomach, she can keep an eye on patients who are vulnerable to becoming anxious. She can forestall an occurrence of anxiety (or at least a severe degree of it), for example, by being available to a patient whose visitors did not arrive, even though they had promised to come. She can expect a patient scheduled for proctoscopy or retrograde pyelography to be nervous not only in relation to the anticipated physical discomfort and the outcome of the procedure, but also in relation to the position he will have to assume in front of his examiners. The nurse can offer to listen to the patient should he wish to ask her questions or should he wish to express some of his thoughts and feelings concerning these matters.

In the same way that the nurse has acquired a certain amount of practice and drill in the handling of physical emergencies, so that she does not have to stop and think when speed and efficiency are required, she could learn to do the same in the area of interpersonal relations.

She can become just as competent in the interpersonal area, as she is now in holding a patient's head in such a way that he will not aspirate his vomitus or in holding the basin in such a way that it will not add extra strain on the already exhausted patient.

For example, she can know exactly how best to relate to a *suspicious* patient; she will not be too friendly with him, not smother him with her attention but rather keep her distance and spell out to him what he is to expect and when.

Similarly she can develop a safe technique in working with *resigned* patients; she will go easy with them, because they cannot tolerate much enthusiasm; she will give them an opportunity to be aware of the warmth of her non-demanding gentleness until they feel the strength to try and want to live once more.

We have touched on various interpersonal techniques throughout the book and shall talk about certain safety measures in the next chapter, but we have not attempted a systematic or exhaustive treatment of this subject matter. In fact, as far as I know, there is no comprehensive treatise covering all the aspects of interpersonal skills in nursing. What is especially needed are definitions of emotional symptoms that are most likely to occur in ourselves and in people under our care, and to make these definitions available to other practitioners in operational form. Then we and they can have easy access to their ingredients and can look for each component and the possible solutions in the actual situation. We need further to test the principles of interpersonal conduct with patients who exhibit certain symptoms and attitudes.

Finally, we need to describe the techniques we are using and have found useful and share them with others, so that they can be tried out by them. If they are found more or less universally valid for nurses, they can be incorporated into our professional body of knowledge.

I see no implicit reason why the nurse cannot attain, through study and supervised practice, in the interpersonal area the competency she has attained in the physical area. As a result she will be just as competent a practitioner in emotional stress, because she will feel secure in what she knows; she will have a *concrete* task to focus on (i.e., her interpersonal techniques) and she will know that she is just as vitally needed by her patients in this area as for physical care. In fact, once she begins to apply her interpersonal skill she will be amazed over and over again at the human needs that lie waiting for expression, and she will be even more surprised at the wealth of human strength that lies dormant behind these needs, waiting to be tapped so it can unfold itself and be transformed into progress and growth.

SUGGESTED READING

Talking with Patients, by Hildegard E. Peplau, in *The American Journal of Nursing*, July 1960.

Chapter **22**
**What the Nurse Can Do
About the Cultural Lag**

In Chapter 4 we said that one of the reasons for a nurse's having "problem" patients lies in the fact that the nurse feels inadequately prepared to deal with sophisticated questions of patients. She does not feel adequately prepared to assume the role of skillful listener which has been delegated to nursing as well as to the other health professions. We discussed helplessness as a state of seeming paralysis resulting from a loss of competency in one area (or a changed situation which results in the impossibility of applying competencies which have worked up till now) and an inability to secure help from the outside to make up for the lack.

In Chapter 18 we talked about ways in which nurses can avoid becoming helpless in the first place, and ways in which they can preserve the competencies that have not been affected by the situation.

In Chapters 19, 20, and 21 we talked of ways in which nurses can cope with frustrations, conflict, and anxiety so that they will not have to resort to becoming helpless.

Now it is time to take a final look at how, under existing circumstances and in light of future demands on her profession, a nurse can acquire the interpersonal competencies (and outside help) that she needs, so she will not be overwhelmed by feelings of inadequacy whenever a patient opens his mouth but can hope to utilize every encounter with him as a meaningful experience for both.

I think that young practitioners, who more likely than not have had some training in interpersonal skills and yet not enough to function independently, must be aware of this aspect of their helplessness. So must many of their older supervisors, who for lack of training cannot provide the supervision which both they and the practitioner know should be given. Both parties avoid the topic, the young nurse in order not to put her superior on the spot (and thus risk a face-saving reprimand from her) and the supervisor in order to keep up appearances. Yet together they could solve some of the problems, if only they felt free to acknowledge each other's strengths and weaknesses: the older person's experience in living and her resulting wisdom (in spite of the lack of theory concerning interpersonal skills), and the younger person's theoretical knowledge of human relations despite her relative lack of sophistication in matters of living.

Unless we do something about alleviating this feeling of inadequacy and helplessness (with a resulting breakdown of communications among staff members as well as between staff and patients), I believe, anxiety, suspicion, and profound discontent will assume such proportions in our hospitals that the resulting climate may seriously affect the progress of patients. We must change nursing curricula to prepare our future nurses better for our rapidly changing times. We must discard the idea that in-service education is a luxury to be extended to nurses as an inducement to come and work in a certain institution. We must accept the fact that it *is* an important part of nursing practice, and that the time required for it, though perhaps taken away from bedside care, is time well invested that will produce rich dividends.

It is my impression that there is little reluctance in setting up in-service programs which have to do with procedures connected with technical advances. But when it comes to developing interpersonal relationship skills, there just never seems to be enough time to devote to this matter or enough money to secure skilled resource people (see also

Chapter 15) . I am not sure what the reason for this hesitancy is, but I think that it has to do with doubts of nurses themselves and others as to whether nurses should assume a listener role. These doubts continue in spite of the recommendations of the Joint Commission on Mental Health and Mental Illness (1) and in spite of the fact that the nurse is the *only* profesional who is in the unique position to assume this listener role on an informal basis day in and day out, without having to subject the patient to the awkward and sometimes frightening process of scheduled listening sessions on a formal basis. I think the reluctance to provide or attend in-service programs that have to do with nurse-patient relationships and listening skills also has to do with the fact that people tend to prefer to improve and enlarge upon those areas of their knowledge in which they already feel reasonably secure, rather than to have to expose their lack of knowledge in areas where they feel rather awkward. And yet, just because of the increased mechanization and complexity of our society, greater demands will be made on people's ability to preserve themselves as living entities in a world of mass production, mass media, mass tastes, and mass expectations of behavior; hence people's need for services to help them find themselves and be themselves will greatly increase (2). Unless the nurse bravely faces her inadequacy in interpersonal relationship skills, which she has not been able to develop, through no fault of her own, and takes a stand for making her contribution in this area as a member of the healing professions, and therefore insists that the necessary preparation and on-going consultation be provided in this area, she is, in my opinion, seriously neglecting her professional obligation.

I am familiar with the frequent objection that it is impossible for nurses to attend in-service meetings or even to set up such meetings because there is such a shortage of staff that the nurses just cannot be spared. This objection is as fallacious as it is common, for one of the reasons for the nurse shortage is that so many women find nursing to be nothing but harassing drudgery and with so little opportunity to learn that they might as well go into other professions or let themselves be supported by their husbands. But the work has become the drudgery it is because the nurse has not had the opportunity to take the time out to learn that (when not too overwhelming) it can be different: rewarding, useful, and self-fulfilling.

Also, people often have an attitude of sacredness about customs, as for instance the eight-hour day. True, it has become a convention to work eight hours in hospitals ever since the Great Depression, but the reason for this was not so much that it was considered to be the optimum amount of time for a nurse to be on the ward with patients, but rather to give a third nurse a chance to earn a share of the then scarce income, heretofore shared by only two nurses. We do not know yet how long a span of time a nurse should spend at the bedside to be of maximum benefit to patients without, at the same time, depleting her inner resources. I think that there are gross individual differences among nurses, and that there are differences relative to the kind of patient they take care of and the demands he or the nature of his condition make on their resources.

But I think that this matter of interpersonal skills should be given careful consideration in the staffing of hospitals, for if it is not, nurses will have to continue to withdraw from the bedside, so they can protect and preserve themselves. Of course, the more inadequate a nurse feels in helping patients to cope with their problems of living, the more she will tend to shun patient contact, in order to protect herself from the devastating feelings of helplessness and guilt for not being able to do more. In order to somehow account for the time they get paid for, these nurses often find themselves cutting out paper labels for chart covers, copying cardex notes, or cleaning endless rows of medicine bottles.

Would it not be more useful if nurses were allowed to spend this time in the hospital library or at in-service discussions, so that with increased knowledge and confidence they could devote more and more productive time to their patients? But who has heard of a staff nurse visiting a library while she is on duty? Doctors may do so, and should, of course; but nurses are to keep up with the literature on their own time. Yet they more than anybody (except, perhaps, for the badly exhausted interns and residents) need their time off duty to replenish their inner resources so that they can go on giving of themselves in such large measure day in and day out.

I do not know what administrators think of such suggestions. I know that to them a hospital is frequently just another kind of industry or business. But even so, they will find much better returns for their investment in the nurse's service if they help to provide the necessary tools to make her work satisfying and worth while for her. How this should be done would be up to the nurses, since it is up to them to set the standards for their work and education (see also Chapter 12). But there is no doubt in my mind that the institution which offers fruitful in-service programs and satisfying workloads will have less worry about turn-over of nurses (3).

What is the nurse to do in the interim? She must continue to function and cannot wait until she has an advanced degree or until hospital circumstances have become more ideal. As I have suggested elsewhere (Chapter 15), it will help if the nurse keeps a log of all problem situations she encounters, and tries to set up clinical conferences in her local nursing organizations in which these problems can be discussed.

It will help also if she attends clinical sessions at national conferences and contributes to them actively by participating in the discussions or by presenting papers on the problems that interest her. Since traveling is expensive, it seems to me that the nurses can rightfully demand some financial aid for such trips from their institutions. For it is not only the nurses who benefit from the gathering of new insights, but also undoubtedly the patients in the hospital. It is patients who are the reason for any health agency's existence.

But what is the nurse to do before she has learned something in the conferences and meetings, provided she is able to attend? She avoids giving patients a chance to unburden themselves to her, because she is afraid they will say more than she can handle, or that she will say the wrong thing and thus hurt them more than they have been hurt already.

Her point is well taken, but I do not think she needs to worry too much; for the chances are slight that if she means well, she can hurt the patient any more than his life experiences have already hurt him. Besides, there are a few basic safety rules, which can tide the nurse over until she gets the necessary supervision.*

First of all, if a patient says something to you that makes you very uncomfortable, you need to examine your discomfort.

Is it because you are setting impossible goals for yourself? Do you feel you *must* find a solution for his problem, and therefore are rather helpless? Relax, if you can; it is not you, it is *he* who must find the solution. You can only help him find it by listening to him, but you cannot do it for him.

Or are you uncomfortable because the patient is disagreeing with something which is of high value to you, for instance, your belief in his doctor? Try to remember that he is not your friend whom you would like to get over on your side, but your patient who is entitled to your help to become clear about himself. What this self is like need not concern you.

Finally, are you uncomfortable because his words or behavior are in some strange way disquieting? If this is the case, do trust your hunch (in fact, always trust your hunches) that something is wrong somewhere. Excuse yourself briefly

* These rules generally follow what I have learned from Hildegard Peplau.

and make sure someone more expert than you takes a look at this patient. Until this someone else comes, you had better stay with the patient and just listen.

And how does one just listen? I think it is a good basic rule, during the first few talks with each patient, to let *him* take the lead in the conversation rather than to structure the talk around your questions with the exception, of course, when you have to find out about his physical condition. If the patient is not saying anything, you can assess the silence for what it appears to be: does he seem afraid of you, or annoyed with you? Does he seem to be trying to think of what to say, or is he deeply preoccupied? Is he in pain? It is best to wait out the silence until you have a pretty good idea of what it is probably all about.

If by then the patient still has not talked, you may ask him about the silence (e.g., "A penny for your thoughts" or "You seem in pain—are you?" "You look puzzled . . ." and so forth). If there seems a blank between you and the patient, be reasonably sure that the blank is not due to your own feeling of awkwardness; if it seems to you that it is, concentrate on your task a little longer until you feel more comfortable. If you feel comfortable enough, you may wish to broach the topic of the patient's present state as compared to his life before he was hospitalized. (There are various examples of this throughout Part II—see Chapter 8, for instance, or Chapter 14). This little technique brings the patient back from wherever he may have been to where he is now, and it puts him and you on a common plane. But do guard yourself from just asking any question in order to get a conversation going. (It is all right to say "Good morning," or "How are things today?" but do not go any further.)

There are two reasons for this. First, you will get merely answers to your questions and remain in the dark as to what is on the patient's mind. Second, you really do not know the patient well, and your question may hit at some area in him which had better be left alone. (For example, you ask

him, "Do you have any children?" and later on you find out
that not only does he not have any but the fact that he was
sterile led his wife to go off with another man.) But that does
not mean you should never ask any questions. A little later
in this chapter we shall discuss what kinds of questions
you can safely ask and when.

If it is you who initiate the conversation by stating that
his hospitalization must be quite a change from the patient's
previous way of life,* you do not spell out what change,
because you do not know. If you guess wrong, you may make
it hard for him to contradict you. If you guess right, he will
think you can read his mind and will either be afraid to
speak, for fear you can always do that, or he will decline to
say much, for why should he make the effort if you can do
it for him.

Suppose the patient says to you, "My wife came yesterday
and brought me some apples." Which of these words are you
supposed to hook on to? "My wife" or "yesterday" or "came"
or "brought" or "apples"? Or are you supposed to say "How
nice?" It is really not complicated. Since you do not have
any idea what the patient is driving at, you do not pick up
any one of the words but rather make some general comment
indicating that you have heard him, that you are interested,
and that he should feel free to go on—something like "oh,"
or "did she?" or "yes?" But do not always use the same
phrase, because the patient will notice this before long and
will beome amused at your obvious show of technique.
"How nice" is a cliché we often use with people whom we
know well, for with them we have some idea what it means
to them. We also use clichés more or less unthinkingly because they underscore what is expected behavior in our society. But now you are neither in a friend's nor in a social
role, but rather in the role of a professional person who

---

* I would not use this technique in a psychiatric hospital, however, because there the illness and the patient as a person are too closely knit together.

makes her services available to her patient so that he can come to grips with his present situation in light of his total life situation. Besides you may be glad you did not say, "how nice" in response to his statement about his wife's visit, because now that he has assessed your neutrality as a listener, he ventures forth with: "Oh yes, and we had a terrible argument." You still do not know what to hook on to, so you can make another noncommittal remark or nod your head for him to continue. After he has supplied you with various additional facts, so that you begin to see a rough outline of the situation, you can ask more specific questions to get a further description of what happened.

Your questions are to help you and the patient to get as complete a picture as possible of the event and its surrounding circumstances. And in order to elicit such a description you can ask questions about what, when, where, or "What happened first?" and "Then what happened?" Because nurses are told they should not start out asking questions of the patient, they are frequently under the misapprehension that they are never to ask any questions. But if you do not ask for further description after the patient has given you a few facts, he will get the impression that you are not interested, since you make no move to draw him out. He will soon change the subject and talk about the weather, or he will fall into a tired (frustrated) silence.

If you have asked questions to elicit further information and the patient still changes the subject, you are getting an indication that this topic is too painful for him at the moment. Make note of the fact in your own mind, but do not force the topic on him. He will get to it when he is ready to do so.

There is one question which you should not ask for quite some time, and that is the question "Why?" The patient does not know the answer to this question; if he did, he would not need to talk to you. If you ask him for a reason and he does not know, he will have to make one up. This helps neither him nor you, really.

When can you ask "why" questions? After the patient has not only given you a full description of the event in question, but has also described to you, upon your encouraging him to do so, at least one but preferably several similar events and has put each step in each event into some kind of time sequence (see the conversation between nurse and patient in Chapter 9). For when the patient gets to this point in his narrative, the reason becomes almost self-evident. For example: "I was anxious, therefore I did not see where I was going" or "I was so angry that I yelled at the first person that came my way—only unfortunately it was my boss."

When the patient reaches the understanding of the reason of his action, you have reached the first landmark of your interviews. This can take anywhere from an hour (with a patient and a nurse who have had a great deal of experience with such talks) to thirty hours, or even longer. If you only have had brief contacts with your patient for only a few days, you may never get to this point with him.

Would it be better, then, not to have talked with him at all? I do not think so. For if you have proceeded safely (i.e., followed slowly the patient's lead instead of following your own curiosity) and have not gone faster than he could go himself (i.e., you have respected his change of subject or his wish to stop the discussion at any point, and you have made yourself available for these talks rather than pushed him into them), you have every reason to assume that the patient was able to handle whatever discoveries he has made until the point of your separation. If he is able to or so inclined, he may use your method of inquiry on his own and talk things over with himself, as it were. If this is not possible, the next person who is in a similar position with him will reap the benefits of your discussion and will be able to proceed that much faster with the patient.

Suppose you are in a position to continue the talks with the patient yourself. What happens after the first landmark is reached, i.e., at the point where you and the patient know that he reacted in a certain way (or became ill) after he was anxious or frustrated or whatever it was. (The more concepts of this kind that you know and their integral components, the better off you are; because this knowledge will enable you to ask the questions which are now necessary to help the patient to recognize, understand, and modify his behavior so he will not have to get into similar difficulties in the future.)

First, you name the concept and ask the patient whether that is what he meant. For example, "You were really in conflict over what you should have done first?" If the patient says yes (if he says no, you just have to listen further to him), you suggest to him that you look together at what conflict really means, just as we did in the various chapters in Part I. Then you can correlate with him the abstract meaning of each step contained in conflict (i.e., the two goals, the movement toward the goals, etc., with the steps he took in the real situation). You can ask him about possible alternatives (i.e., what else might you have done? Given two equal goals, what other manipulations were possible?). And by then he has surely caught on and is probably pleased as Punch with the new tool you have given him. But before you leave him completely to his joy, you will need to make sure that he really has learned to recognize the concept in question for what it is (i.e., the symptoms by which it manifests itself, in the case of conflict—hesitation, vacillation, indecisiveness, and fatigue). For it does not help to know a solution when one does not know when to apply it.

There is much more to be said about talking with patients that is beyond the scope of this book.

I would like to conclude with two brief warnings.

First, although my suggestions of how to talk with patients will probably keep you within safe and reasonable practice, they do not substitute for the supervision you need and are entitled to and should get before too long.

Second, patients are not used to the fact that nurses may know how to listen to them. And as a result, some of them may become a little anxious and suspicious about the way you listen. Some of them may even "accuse" you of playing psychiatrist or trying to sound them out for secrets. This is hard to take, especially when one means well and when one knows that one is just performing the job one is supposed to perform.

I think it may help if you can explore with the patient what it is that you have done or said that reminds him of a psychiatrist. You can also agree with him, after he tells you, that there are some points in common in all professional listening; but a psychiatrist's task is quite different from that of a nurse. A psychiatrist usually helps a patient to change his personality, or at least some of its attributes, so that he can cope better with his life. A nurse's goals are less ambitious (unless she is a trained psychiatric nurse specialist): she aims at helping the patient to take stock of himself in a particular life situation (in the hospital it may be the fact of his hospitalization) and how this might relate to some of his habitual patterns of living. She aims further at helping him to examine these particular patterns of living as to their usefulness in coping with his life in general and their effectiveness in keeping him well.

If, after this explanation, the patient is still suspicious, you can let him know squarely that you are available to talk to him but that it is up to him to take you up on your offer. The more squarely you deal with your patients, the easier it will be for you to cope with suspiciousness should it arise, and also the more trust a patient will develop. Thus, let him know early that the focus of the relationship is on him, since it is a professional relationship for his benefit. Let him know also at the beginning of your talks how often and when and for how long he can expect to talk with you, and who will be informed about the content of your talks. The only time when you may have to let other (than previously stated) people know about the confidential content of your talk will be if the patient mentions intentions of self-destruction or if he has any physical complaints which are not known to his doctor. In either of these cases you must tell the patient that either you or he or both of you will have to report this matter, and you will have to stay with him until it is reported.

I think that once you have gotten into the habit of "listening" to patients along the lines we have suggested in this book, and once you have had the opportunity for the necessary supervision and the learning of additional skill in this area, you will soon feel less helpless, therefore less defensive, when confronted by difficult behavior on the part of your patients. Who knows, before long you will not have any problem patients, only challenging situations which are beckoning to you to try to resolve them.

Suggested Reading

Several articles by Hildegard E. Peplau, in *The American Journal of Nursing*:
Loneliness, December 1955;
Themes in Nursing Situations, October and November 1953;
Utilizing Themes in Nursing Situations, March 1954.
Personal, Impersonal and Interpersonal Relations by Genevieve Burton (Springer, 1958).
Interviewing, Its Methods and Techniques by Annette Garrett (Family Service Association, New York, 1942).
Talking With Patients by Brian Bird (Lippincott, 1955).
Therapeutic Communication by Jurgen Ruesch (Norton, 1961).
The Technique of Psychotherapy by Lewis Robert Wolberg (Grune & Stratton, 1954).

NOTES ON SOURCES

INTRODUCTION

1. Cathleen Cockburn and Gertrud Ujhely, *A Study to Determine Areas in Nurse-Patient Relationships Where Nurses Need Help*. Unpublished paper, Teachers College, Columbia University, New York, 1956.

2. Betty Harmuth, Ura Lantz, and Gloria Oden, *The Problem Patient*. Unpublished paper, Rutgers, The State University of New Jersey, Newark, N.J., 1961.

3. Catherine M. Norris, The Nurse and the Dying Patient, *The American Journal of Nursing*, 55:10 (October 1955), pp. 1214-16.

4. ———, The Nurse and the Crying Patient, *The American Journal of Nursing*, 57:3 (March 1957), pp. 323-27.

5. Morris Schwartz and Emmy Lanning Schockley, *The Nurse and the Mental Patient: A Study in Interpersonal Relations*. New York: Russell Sage Foundation, 1956.

CHAPTER 1

1. David Fox and others, *Career Decisions and Professional Expectations of Nursing Students*. New York: Teachers College, Columbia University, 1961.

CHAPTER 3

1. Hildegard E. Peplau, *A Working Definition of Anxiety*. Unpublished paper.

CHAPTER 4

1. Victor E. Frankl, *From Death Camp to Existentialism*. Boston: Beacon Press, 1959.

CHAPTER 8

1. Bertrand Russell, *The Conquest of Happiness*, London: Allen, 1961.

CHAPTER 9

1. Wilhelm Reich, *Character Analysis*, 3rd ed., Rangeley, Maine: Orgone Institute Press, 1949.

CHAPTER 12

1. Genevieve Bixler and Roy Bixler, The Professional Status of Nursing, *The American Journal of Nursing, 59*:8, pp. 1142-47.

CHAPTER 15

1. Theodore Lidz, General Concepts of Psychosomatic Medicine, in *American Handbook of Psychiatry,* edited by Silvano Arieti, Vol. I. New York: Basic Books, 1959.

2. Edward Weiss and O. Spurgeon English, *Psychosomatic Medicine,* 3rd ed., Philadelphia: Saunders, 1957.

3. Roy Grinker and Fred P. Robbins, *Psychosomatic Case Book.* New York: The Blakiston Co., 1954.

4. Leo W. Simmons and Harold Wolff, *Social Science in Medicine.* New York: Russell Sage Foundation, 1954.

5. Wilhelm Reich, *The Discovery of the Orgone*: Vol II, *The Cancer Biopathy.* Rangeley, Maine: Orgone Institute Press, 1948.

6. Harold G. Wolff, *Stress and Disease.* Springfield, Ill.: Charles C Thomas, 1953.

7. Goldie Ruth Kabak, *Survey of Student Opinions About Learning Experiences.* New York: National League for Nursing. 1960.

8. Joint Commission on Mental Health and Mental Illness, *Action for Mental Health.* New York: Basic Books, 1961.

CHAPTER 19

1. Frances Reiter, The Improvement of Nursing Practice, in *Improvement of Nursing Practice.* New York: American Nurses' Association, 1961.

2. Victor E. Frankl, *The Doctor and the Soul.* New York: Knopf, 1955.

CHAPTER 20

1. David Riesman, *The Lonely Crowd.* New York: Doubleday, 1953.

2. Bruno Bettelheim, *The Informed Heart.* Glencoe, Ill.: The Free Press, 1960.

CHAPTER 22

1. Joint Commission on Mental Health and Mental Illness, *Action for Mental Health.* New York: Basic Books, 1961.

2. Bruno Bettelheim, *The Informed Heart.* Glencoe, Ill.: The Free Press, 1960.

INDEX